This page is intentionally left blank

Medical Disclaimer

The information provided in this book is for educational and informational purposes only and is not intended as medical advice. The content is not intended to be a substitute for professional medical advice, diagnosis, or treatment. Always seek the advice of your physician or other qualified health providers with any questions you may have regarding a medical condition. The authors and publishers of this book have made every effort to ensure that the information contained herein is accurate and reliable.

However, the information is provided "as is" without warranty of any kind, either express or implied, and the authors and publishers make no representations or warranties regarding its completeness, accuracy, reliability, suitability, or availability. Any reliance you place on such information is therefore strictly at your own risk.

The authors and publishers shall not be held responsible or liable for any loss, injury, or damage allegedly arising from any information or suggestions in this book. No doctor patient relationship is formed. Readers are encouraged to confirm the information contained herein with other sources and to consult with a qualified healthcare professional before making any medical or health-related decisions based on the content of this book.

In the event of a medical emergency, call a doctor or 911 immediately. Do not disregard or delay seeking professional medical advice because of something you have read in this book.

By using this book, you agree to these terms and conditions. If you do not agree with these terms and conditions, you should not use this book.

Table of Contents

Introduction
By: Jonathan Kahan MD

What is cardiovascular disease?

Cardiovascular disease (CVD) encompasses a range of conditions affecting the heart and blood vessels, including coronary artery disease, stroke, hypertension (high blood pressure), congestive heart failure, atherosclerosis, high cholesterol, and peripheral arterial disease [1].

Why do we care about cardiovascular disease (CVD)?

Cardiovascular disease is the number one killer in the world by far. Annually, approximately 18 million people die of cardiovascular disease. If you added up the next 10 leading causes including all cancers (12 million annual deaths) it would not equal CVD death for that year. There are 60% more cardiovascular deaths today than there were in 1990 per capita. One person in the US dies every 34 seconds from cardiovascular disease. At the height of the COVID 19 pandemic, 250% more people died of CVD then from COVID. Thirty five percent of all acute myocardial infarctions (heart attacks) occur at the age of 30-55 years old. Forty eight percent of women > 20 years old have some evidence of CVD. Only 6.8% of US adults were optimal for cardiometabolic health in 2022, and this number is worsening [2-6].

What percentage of cardiovascular disease is preventable?

Ninety (90%)!

How do we prevent cardiovascular disease?

By following the advice in this book and working with your physician. It breaks down into a discussion of two broad categories:

<table>
<tr><td align="center"><u>**Prevention:**</u></td><td align="center"><u>**Health/Resilience:**</u></td></tr>
<tr><td align="center">Smoking
High Blood Pressure
Cholesterol</td><td align="center">Obesity and Diet
Exercise
Sleep
Social/Miscellaneous</td></tr>
</table>

What does primary prevention mean? What does health mean? Why are we escaping history?

Primary prevention: to prevent a disease before it occurs, specifically in this case cardiovascular diseases [7].

Health: The World Health Organization (WHO) defines "Health" as a state of <u>complete physical, mental and social well-being and not merely the absence of disease or infirmity</u> [8]. As the WHO states, it is not just about absence of disease, but an all-encompassing wellbeing. The tools in this book will help make you healthy.

Escaping History: In this book you will be given the skills to escape your personal and your family's cardiovascular history. Early family history of cardiovascular disease (CVD) is defined as a diagnosis of CVD in an immediate male relative less than 55 years old or a female immediate relative less than 65 years old (parents or siblings). Individuals with an early family history of cardiovascular disease are at 70% increased risk of developing heart disease themselves! We will teach you how to escape this fate. Furthermore, your personal history of obesity, metabolic dysfunction, smoking, poor diet, sleep, mood and physical condition will be transformed as well. You are not who you were yesterday, and it is time to become the best version of you possible!

References

1. Thiriet M. Cardiovascular Disease: An Introduction. *Biomathematical and Biomechanical Modeling of the Circulatory and Ventilatory Systems*. 2018;8(PMC7123129):1-90. doi:https://doi.org/10.1007/978-3-319-89315-0_1
2. World Health Organization. Cardiovascular diseases (CVDs). World Health Organization. Published June 11, 2021. https://www.who.int/news-room/fact-sheets/detail/cardiovascular-diseases-(cvds)
3. World Heart Federation. Deaths from cardiovascular disease surged 60% globally over the last 30 years: Report. World Heart Federation. Published May 20, 2023. https://world-heart-federation.org/news/deaths-from-cardiovascular-disease-surged-60-globally-over-the-last-30-years-report/
4. More than half of U.S. adults don't know heart disease is leading cause of death, despite 100-year reign. American Heart Association. Accessed May 7, 2024. https://newsroom.heart.org/news/more-than-half-of-u-s-adults-dont-know-heart-disease-is-leading-cause-of-death-despite-100-year-reign#:~:text=There%20are%202%2C552%20deaths%20from%20total%20cardiovascular%20disease
5. Cardiovascular deaths saw steep rise in U.S. during first year of the COVID-19 pandemic. www.heart.org. https://www.heart.org/en/news/2023/01/25/cardiovascular-deaths-saw-steep-rise-in-us-during-first-year-of-the-covid-19-pandemic
6. Gulati R, Behfar A, Narula J, et al. Acute Myocardial Infarction in Young Individuals. *Mayo Clinic Proceedings*. 2020;95(1):136-156. doi:https://doi.org/10.1016/j.mayocp.2019.05.001
7. Kisling L, Das J. Prevention Strategies. National Library of Medicine. Published August 1, 2023. https://www.ncbi.nlm.nih.gov/books/NBK537222/
8. Schramme T. Health as Complete Well-Being: The WHO Definition and Beyond. *Public Health Ethics*. 2023;16(3). doi:https://doi.org/10.1093/phe/phad017

Smoking/Vaping/Marijuana

By: Valeria Ramirez Lombana MD, Muhammad Adnan Haider MD, Jonathan Kahan MD

What you need to know

1. Smoking directly leads to cardiovascular disease such as heart attacks and strokes. You do not realize how sick you are until you finally stop for good!
2. Quitting smoking at any age is one of the best things you can do for your health
3. There are multiple effective tools to help quit smoking. Using a tool to help quit smoking increases your chances over cold turkey
4. The average smoker attempts to quit at least 6 times before quitting permanently, do not give up!

Smoking has evolved into a widespread social habit over centuries, deeply intertwined with cultural, economic, and social aspects of societies around the world. However, it is now known to have profound implications for public health. Aside from the well documented association with respiratory ailments and cancer, smoking is the number one modifiable risk factor for cardiovascular disease. As of today, 11% of adults aged 18-24 vape, 17% of US adults use vape/smoked marijuana and 11.5% of adults smoke cigarettes/tobacco. These numbers are increasing in every category annually [1].

What are modifiable risk factors?

These are factors that individuals can change or influence through lifestyle choices or medical treatment. For example: smoking, physical inactivity, unhealthy diet, obesity, high blood pressure, high cholesterol, and diabetes.

What are non-modifiable risk factors?

These factors are beyond individual control and cannot be altered. They include age, race, and genetic predisposition. For instance, the risk of CVD increases with age, and men are at a higher risk at a younger age compared to women, though the risk for women increases and can surpass that of men as they age.

Why is smoking bad?

Smoking is a leading cause of CVD-related morbidity and mortality, responsible for a substantial proportion of preventable deaths worldwide. The detrimental effects of smoking on cardiovascular health involve mechanisms such as oxidative stress, inflammation, endothelial dysfunction, and alterations in lipid metabolism [2].

What is oxidative stress?

Oxidative stress occurs when there's an imbalance between the production of free radicals (reactive oxygen species or ROS) and the body's ability to detoxify these reactive products or repair the resulting damage. Cigarette smoke contains a high concentration of free radicals and other reactive oxygen species. When inhaled, these substances can overwhelm the body's antioxidant defenses, leading to cellular damage. This damage is a result of the oxidation of cellular components like lipids (see cholesterol section), proteins, and DNA, which can lead to various diseases, including cardiovascular diseases, cancer, and chronic obstructive pulmonary disease (COPD) [3].

How does smoking cause inflammation?

Cigarette smoke can trigger an inflammatory response in the body. The chemicals in smoke activate immune cells, such as macrophages and neutrophils, leading to the production of inflammatory cytokines and mediators. This chronic inflammatory state not only damages tissues but also promotes the progression of atherosclerosis (the buildup of fats, cholesterol, and other substances in and on the artery walls) as well as other inflammatory diseases. The persistent inflammation can further exacerbate oxidative stress, creating a vicious cycle that contributes to disease progression [4].

What is endothelial dysfunction?

The endothelium is the thin layer of cells lining the inside of blood vessels, playing a key role in maintaining vascular health by regulating blood pressure and blood flow, and preventing clotting. Smoking can cause endothelial dysfunction, which is an early and critical step in the development of atherosclerosis (plaque or blockages in the arteries). The chemicals in cigarette smoke can damage the endothelium, leading to reduced production of nitric oxide (NO), a molecule essential for vasodilation (the widening of blood vessels). Additionally, the oxidative stress and inflammation induced by smoking further impair endothelial function. This dysfunction promotes the development of plaques in the arteries, leading to cardiovascular diseases such as heart attacks, strokes, erectile dysfunction, peripheral artery disease [5,6].

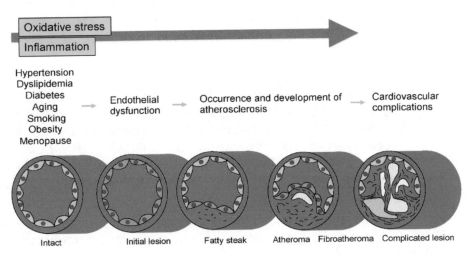

Higashi Y. Roles of Oxidative Stress and Inflammation in Vascular Endothelial Dysfunction-Related Disease. *Antioxidants*. 2022;11(10):1958. doi:https://doi.org/10.3390/antiox11101958

How does smoking affect lipid (cholesterol) metabolism?

Smoking affects lipid metabolism in several ways, leading to unfavorable changes in blood lipid profiles. It can increase the levels of low-density lipoprotein (LDL) cholesterol (often referred to as "bad" cholesterol) and decrease levels of high-density lipoprotein (HDL) cholesterol ("good" cholesterol). This alteration in lipid levels contributes to the development of atherosclerosis. The mechanisms behind these changes include oxidative modifications of

9

lipoproteins, alterations in the activity of enzymes involved in lipid metabolism, and changes in the liver's metabolism of lipids. These lipid profile changes further elevate the risk of cardiovascular diseases [7].

What are the different types of smoking?

1. Cigarettes: Traditional cigarettes consist of dried tobacco leaves wrapped in paper, often containing various additives. Combustion of tobacco generates a complex mixture of toxic compounds, including tar, carbon monoxide, heavy metals and numerous carcinogens. Regular cigarette smoking is strongly associated with an increased risk of CVD, with long-term exposure exacerbating arterial plaque formation, thrombosis, and endothelial dysfunction. Note menthol cigarettes are even worse than regular, as they mask any inhalation pain leading to increased inhalation, and contain other additives which are carcinogenic [8].

2. Light Cigarettes: Marketed as a 'healthier' alternative, light cigarettes typically contain lower levels of tar. However, smokers of light cigarettes often compensate by smoking more intensely or inhaling deeper, negating any potential benefits. Additionally, there are larger holes in the filter of light cigarettes, which are covered with fingers anyways when a cigarette is held, again negating any positive effects. Studies suggest that light cigarettes confer a similar risk of CVD as regular cigarettes, with no significant cardiovascular advantages.

3. Vaping (Electronic Cigarettes): Electronic cigarettes, or e-cigarettes (ecig), have emerged as a popular alternative to traditional smoking. These devices heat a liquid solution (e-liquid) containing nicotine, flavorings, and other chemicals, producing an aerosol that users inhale. Despite being promoted as a safer alternative, the long-term cardiovascular effects of vaping are still not understood. Emerging evidence suggests potential adverse effects on endothelial function, arterial stiffness, and platelet aggregation, raising concerns about their cardiovascular safety. Long term data is lacking in many cases. However, they are also emerging as a tool to

temporarily quit regular cigarettes (see below). Note "popcorn lung" (broncholitis obliterans) is actually from diacetyl in flavored ecig/vape and should be avoided.

4. Alternative Forms of Tobacco: Among these products are **cigars,** which are tobacco wrapped in leaf tobacco or another tobacco-containing substance, and **cigarillos,** smaller cigars that are generally cheaper and can be bought individually. **Hookahs or waterpipes** are another popular option, where smoke is drawn through a long, flexible tube and filtered through water before inhalation. **Smokeless tobacco**, like chewing tobacco and snuff, is used by placing the product between the teeth and gums, offering a smoke-free experience. Additionally, there's **powder tobacco,** a mixture that is inhaled through the nose. All carry similar risks as traditional forms of tobacco use.

5. Secondhand and Thirdhand smoking: Secondhand smoke, also known as passive or secondary smoke, poses a significant public health risk. It is linked to a 20% increase in lung cancer risk among nonsmokers and is estimated to cause around 53,800 deaths annually in the United States Moreover, exposure to secondhand smoke at home is a risk factor for childhood asthma. [9] Thirdhand smoke, a lesser-known concern, refers to the chemical residue left on surfaces after smoking. These residues can persist long after the smoke has dissipated, posing a risk to anyone who might touch, inhale or ingest them.

6. Cannabis (marijuana/weed smoking/vaping): The cardiovascular effects of smoking cannabis are not as extensively studied as tobacco, but research indicates several potential risks. Cannabis smoking has been associated with an increased heart rate, fluctuations in blood pressure, and a potential increase in the risk of heart attack and stroke, especially in individuals with pre-existing heart conditions. The combustion products inhaled when smoking cannabis can also harm the cardiovascular system similarly to tobacco smoke, although frequency of use appears to be less than traditional tobacco.

Note: Regardless of the form, smoking exerts detrimental effects on every organ system, contributing to a variety of health conditions beyond CVD. Chronic smoking is associated with an increased risk of respiratory infections, chronic obstructive pulmonary disease (COPD), cancer (lung, throat, esophagus, etc.), and various metabolic disorders. Moreover, exposure to secondhand smoke poses a significant health threat, particularly for nonsmokers, increasing the risk of CVD and respiratory illnesses [10].

What is the prevalence of Tobacco, Nicotine and E-Cigarettes use in the USA?

Quitting smoking is crucial for your health, given the high prevalence of tobacco use. According to the National Institute on Drug Abuse, in 2021, about 22% of people aged 12 or older reported using tobacco products or vaping nicotine in the past 30 days, equating to 61.6 million people. Of these, 15.6% (43.6 million people) smoked cigarettes, and 4.7% (13.2 million people) vaped nicotine in the last month.

Among young students, the trend is concerning. In 2022, about 8.7% of 8th graders, 15.1% of 10th graders, and 24.8% of 12th graders reported using nicotine in the past 30 days. The numbers for cigarette use were lower, with 0.8% of 8th graders, 1.7% of 10th graders, and 4% of 12th graders reporting use. However, vaping nicotine was notably higher, with 7.1% of 8th graders, 14.2% of 10th graders, and 20.7% of 12th graders reporting vaping in the past 30 days [11]

Improving Cardiovascular Health: Quitting Smoking

It's never too late to quit smoking. Quitting smoking is the most effective action you can take to enhance your cardiovascular health and overall well-being (other than increasing VO2Max, see exercise section). Smoking is a major risk factor for cardiovascular disease (CVD) and stopping can significantly lower your risk of heart disease, stroke, and other health complications. By quitting, you not only improve your own health but also reduce the risk of secondhand smoke exposure for those around you. The Surgeon General's Report on Smoking Cessation, released in January 2020, confirms that quitting smoking is beneficial at any age. It improves health, reduces the risk of early death, and can add up to ten years to your life. This is why physicians are encouraged to provide support for quitting to both young people and parents who smoke. Methods which can help quitting:

1. Electronic Cigarettes
2. Behavior Counseling
3. Nicotine Replacement Therapies
4. Prescription Medications
5. Technology Based Interventions

What Are Electronic Cigarettes and Can They Help You Quit Smoking?

Electronic cigarettes (ECs) are small devices that create vapor (or aerosol) by heating a liquid solution, typically containing nicotine and other chemicals. Some smokers turn to ECs to help them quit or cut back on smoking, but their safety and effectiveness are debated. Many healthcare professionals and policymakers are cautious about recommending them due to limited evidence on long-term health impacts. This review update is part of an ongoing effort to assess whether ECs can be used as a smoking cessation tool and if they're safe for regular use.

There is growing evidence that ECs are helping people quit smoking compared to conventional nicotine replacement therapy (gum, patches etc). For example, A review of 78 studies with 22,052 adult smokers found that people are more likely to quit smoking for at least six months using nicotine e-cigarettes compared to other methods like nicotine replacement therapy, varenicline, e-cigarettes without nicotine, or no support. The review showed that for every 100 people using nicotine e-cigarettes, 8 to 12 out of 100 might successfully stop smoking, whereas only 6 of 100 people using nicotine replacement therapy and 7 of 100 using e-cigarettes without nicotine might quit. [12]

In another systematic review examining whether e-cigarettes could help people quit or reduce smoking. Among 7,551 participants across six studies, nicotine-filled e-cigarettes were more effective than those without nicotine, with 18% of 1,242 smokers achieving cessation after at least six months of use. [13].

Compared to regular cigarettes, ECs appear to be safer in terms of heart attacks and strokes. This is likely secondary to larger particle size and not burning organic materials. In the PRISMA review, the odds of having a heart attack were higher in e-cigarettes (e-cigarettes only or e-cigarettes + traditional smoking) users [OR 1.33 (95% CI = 1.14–1.56, p-value = 0.01] in comparison to nonsmokers but significantly less than compared to traditional smokers [OR 0.61 (95% CI = 0.40–0.93, p-value 0.02]. Figure 1 below shows different types of electronic cigarettes.

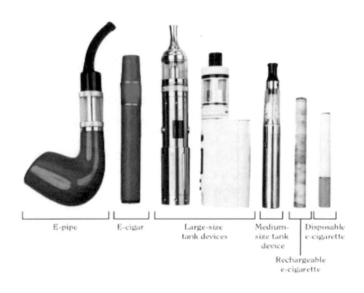

| E-pipe | E-cigar | Large-size tank devices | Medium-size tank device | Disposable e-cigarette |

Rechargeable e-cigarette

[12]

Conventional Methods of Smoking Cessation

After explaining the role of ECs let's discuss the role of some conventional methods of smoking cessation. Quitting smoking is possible with the help of effective treatments that include both counseling and FDA-approved medications. Comparison of the effectiveness of each method is given in **table 1 of the appendix**.

1. **Behavioral Counseling:** Quitting smoking can be tough, but there is help available. Behavioral counseling is a method where you work with specialists to help you quit smoking. These specialists are trained to provide support over several sessions, usually four to eight, to guide you through the quitting process. You can receive this counseling either in person or over the phone, and it's even more effective when

combined with quitting medications. There are different ways to approach counseling, so you can find the one that works best for you. The Affordable Care Act (ACA) changes how health insurance works in the U.S. and focuses more on prevention, including coverage for quitting smoking. The ACA suggests that insurance should cover at least two attempts to quit each year, with four counseling sessions (each lasting at least 10 minutes), and FDA-approved medications for quitting smoking, whether prescribed or over the counter, for a 90-day period. This could make it much easier to get treatment for tobacco addiction, but in reality, not all insurance companies are fully implementing or advertising these benefits. [14, 15] Different forms of behavior therapies are:

I) Cognitive Behavior Therapy (CBT) Cognitive Behavioral Therapy (CBT) helps people understand what makes them want to smoke—like certain people, places, or things—and teaches them ways to avoid giving in to those triggers. CBT offers skills to prevent relapse, like relaxation techniques, and effective ways to handle stress without smoking. Studies show that both CBT and basic health education can help reduce nicotine dependence, but one study found that smokers using nicotine patches who had six sessions of intensive group CBT had higher success rates in quitting than those who had six sessions of general health education. [16, 17]

II) Motivational Interviewing (MI) Motivational Interviewing (MI) is a method where counselors work with you to help you think about why you might be unsure about quitting smoking and to find reasons to make healthier choices. MI is all about you, without any arguments or pressure. The counselor will help you see how your current behavior might not line up with what you really want in life. They listen to your concerns and help you feel more confident and positive about quitting smoking. Studies show that MI can lead to better quit rates than just giving brief advice to stop smoking or providing standard care. [18]

III) Mindfulness-In mindfulness-based smoking cessation treatments, patients are taught to be more aware of their thoughts, feelings, and cravings, without getting caught up in them. This therapy encourages you to pay attention to the thoughts and feelings that might make you want to smoke and to see them as normal and manageable. The goal is to help you deal with stress and cravings without going back to smoking or other unhealthy habits. Over the past decade, more people have shown interest in mindfulness-based treatments, and studies indicate that this approach can improve mental health and reduce the risk of starting to smoke again. However, more studies are needed to better understand its effectiveness. [19]

2. Nicotine Replacement Therapy (NRT)

Nicotine Replacement Therapy (NRT) is available in different forms that you can buy without a prescription. These include patches, sprays, gum, and lozenges, and they all work equally well to help people quit smoking. NRTs provide the brain with a small dose of nicotine to ease withdrawal symptoms and cravings, which can be intense when you stop smoking. Many people use NRTs to help them get through the tough early stages of quitting, and those with stronger nicotine addictions may benefit from longer-term use. Clinical trials of NRT in patients with underlying, stable coronary disease suggest that nicotine does not increase cardiovascular risk. The risks of NRT for smokers, even for those with underlying cardiovascular disease, are small and are substantially outweighed by the potential benefits of smoking cessation. [20]

Research shows that using NRT improves your chances of quitting smoking, and if you add counseling or other behavioral therapies, you're even more likely to succeed. The most effective approach is to combine a steady dose of nicotine from a patch with another form of NRT like gum or lozenges, which you can use as needed when cravings hit. This combination can be better at reducing withdrawal symptoms and cravings than just using one type of NRT. Studies suggest that NRT can boost quit rates by 50 to 70 percent. Using the nicotine patch for up to 24 weeks is considered safe. [21, 22]. **Comparison of different NRT and specific dosing is given in Table 2. of the appendix.**

3. **Prescription Medications:** Several prescription medications, such as bupropion and varenicline, can help reduce nicotine cravings and withdrawal symptoms, enhancing the likelihood of successful cessation.

I) Bupropion

Bupropion, a medication first used to treat depression, can also help people quit smoking. It works by affecting certain brain chemicals, norepinephrine and dopamine, which are linked to mood and motivation. Studies show that people who use bupropion are more likely to quit smoking compared to those who don't take it. This has been proven in both short-term and long-term studies. Bupropion is as effective as nicotine replacement therapy (NRT), making it a useful option for those looking to stop smoking. [23]

II) Varenicline

Varenicline is a medication that can help reduce cravings for nicotine by working on a specific receptor in the brain, but it does this less strongly than actual nicotine. This makes it easier for people to quit smoking because it decreases the urge to smoke. Studies show that people who take varenicline are more likely to quit compared to those who try without any assistance. It has also been shown to be more effective than using just one type of nicotine replacement therapy (NRT) or bupropion.

In a study done in a primary care setting, 44% of people who took varenicline, with or without counseling, were smoke-free after two years. Those who joined group therapy and followed the medication schedule had better results in staying smoke-free. Overall, research suggests that varenicline may be a better option for quitting smoking than bupropion [24]

III) Combination Medications

Combining different medications may help people quit smoking more effectively. Some studies show that using nicotine replacement therapy (NRT) with other medicines can improve success rates. For example, one analysis found that using both varenicline and NRT (like wearing a nicotine patch before quitting) was more effective than using varenicline alone. Similarly, adding bupropion to NRT improved the chances of quitting smoking.

For smokers who had a hard time cutting back with just the NRT patch, using extended-release bupropion with varenicline was more effective than a placebo. This was especially true for men and people who were heavily addicted to nicotine. These combinations offer promising options for those who struggle with quitting. [25]

IV) Other Antidepressant

Besides bupropion, some other antidepressants can also help people quit smoking, even though they're primarily used for treating depression. These medications are considered second-choice options for quitting smoking. A few smaller studies suggest that nortriptyline, an antidepressant, works just as well as nicotine replacement therapy (NRT) to help people quit smoking.

While nortriptyline can have side effects in some patients, the small studies focusing on its use for quitting smoking didn't report any major issues. On the other hand, selective serotonin reuptake inhibitors (SSRIs), which include fluoxetine, paroxetine, and sertraline, don't seem to help people quit smoking, even when combined with NRT. This finding has been consistent in research.

V) Transcranial Magnetic Stimulation

Transcranial magnetic stimulation (TMS) is a new method being tested to help treat addiction. It uses magnetic fields to stimulate certain parts of the brain without surgery or needles. When multiple pulses of TMS are given in a row, it's called repetitive TMS (rTMS). The FDA has approved two rTMS devices for treating depression in adults.

Research on using rTMS to help people quit smoking is still in the early stages, but the results look promising. In studies with adult smokers who couldn't quit using other treatments, high-frequency TMS reduced the number of cigarettes they smoked. When high-frequency TMS was combined with cues that remind people of smoking, it became even more effective, with 44% of participants quitting by the end of treatment. Six months later, 33% of those treated with this method were still smoke-free. More studies with larger groups are needed to confirm how well rTMS works for helping people quit smoking. [26]

4. Technology Based Interventions

I)Text messaging, web-based services, and social media support

Technology like mobile phones and the internet can play a role in helping people quit smoking. These tools make it easier for people to get support, especially if they live far from treatment centers or can't travel easily. Even simple things like getting text messages with quitting tips or using a website for quitting advice can be helpful. Studies have shown that adults who receive support through these methods are more likely to quit smoking than those who don't.

Among adults who call a Quitline for help, most prefer a mix of phone and web-based support instead of just online programs. This combined approach seems to keep people more engaged in their journey to quit. Technology-based programs are also gaining popularity among young adults aged 18 to 25, a group with high smoking rates. Social media has had a largely negative impact on the smoking status of youth (see also social section), especially among teenagers. A study done on teenage users of TikTok found that frequent interaction with tobacco-related content significantly increased the likelihood of e-cigarette use. Teens who used TikTok several times per day or who regularly saw tobacco-related posts were more likely to start using e-cigarettes compared to their peers who engaged less with such content. This underscores the need for careful regulation of tobacco content on social platforms to prevent adverse impacts on youth smoking rates. [27, 28]

Removing smoking advertisements from public view can significantly reduce smoking rates. This idea follows the concept of "out of sight, out of mind." For instance, not displaying smoking scenes or including health warnings about the dangers of smoking in movies, dramas, or shows can help lower the rate of smoking. This approach is supported by evidence from a study in Australia, where bans on displaying tobacco packs at points of sale were implemented. The study found that such bans led to a decrease in young people's recall of tobacco displays, a reduced overestimation of peer smoking rates, lower tobacco brand awareness, and fewer young people smoking. Overall, these bans helped make smoking less normal and appealing among youth. This suggests that reducing the visibility of tobacco in various media and retail settings can be an effective strategy in discouraging smoking among young people and the general population. [29]

II) Telephone support and Quitline

If you're trying to quit smoking, you can call a toll-free Quitline to get help from trained counselors. Every state has a Quitline, and you can reach them at **1-800-QUIT-NOW (1-800-784-8669)**. These Quitlines offer information and support to help you quit smoking. Studies have shown that people who call Quitlines are more likely to succeed in quitting, especially when counselors call them back for multiple sessions. It's not clear exactly how many calls are best, but people who get at least three follow-up calls are more likely to quit than those who only get educational materials or brief advice.

Quitlines aren't just for people who smoke cigarettes; they can also help if you use smokeless tobacco. Another Quitline run by the U.S. Department of Health and Human Services can be reached at **1-877-44U-QUIT (1-877-448-7848)**. If you prefer online resources, you can visit https://smokefree.gov/ for more tools to help you quit smoking, including text message support and other phone-based services. [30]

5. **Support Groups and Peer Networks:** Joining support groups, either in-person or online, can provide individuals with a sense of community and accountability, facilitating mutual encouragement and shared experiences. Peer support networks offer a non-judgmental environment where individuals can seek guidance, share challenges, and celebrate milestones on their cessation journey.[SEP]

6. **Lifestyle Modifications:** Engaging in regular physical activity, adopting stress-reduction techniques (e.g., mindfulness, yoga), and making dietary changes can complement smoking cessation efforts and promote overall cardiovascular health. These healthier habits can help individuals manage cravings, reduce nicotine dependence, and maintain long-term abstinence.[SEP]

7. **Quitting Smoking During Pregnancy**
Smoking during pregnancy is risky, but quitting can be challenging. Many pregnant women want to quit, but they often need support to succeed. Researchers have explored different ways to help pregnant women quit smoking, focusing on behavioral treatments since medications tend to have limited success.

Behavioral counseling combined with incentives like vouchers has proven most effective for pregnant women trying to quit smoking. Offering vouchers along with regular care, which included free nicotine replacement therapy for 10 weeks and four weekly support phone calls, more than doubled the chances of quitting during pregnancy. Studies show that these behavioral approaches reduce preterm births and increase the birth weight of babies compared to regular care. Additionally, incentives like vouchers have been linked to better fetal growth, higher birth weight, fewer low-birth-weight deliveries, and longer breastfeeding periods [31,32]

Smoking is the number one modifiable risk factor for cardiovascular disease, exerting deleterious effects on cardiovascular health through various mechanisms. Understanding the different forms of smoking and their associated health risks is essential for implementing effective prevention and cessation strategies. By promoting smoking cessation and adopting healthier lifestyle behaviors, individuals can significantly reduce their risk of CVD and improve their overall quality of life.

References

1. Products - Data Briefs - Number 475 - July 2023. www.cdc.gov. Published July 28, 2023. https://www.cdc.gov/nchs/products/databriefs/db475.htm#:~:text=Current%20e%2D cigarette%20use%20was
2. Redirecting. linkinghub.elsevier.com. Accessed May 17, 2024. https://linkinghub.elsevier.com/retrieve/pii/000293439290620Q
3. Padmavathi P, Raghu PS, Reddy VD, et al. Chronic cigarette smoking-induced oxidative/nitrosative stress in human erythrocytes and platelets. Molecular & Cellular Toxicology. 2018;14(1):27-34. doi:https://doi.org/10.1007/s13273-018-0004-6
4. Wang H, Chen H, Fu Y, et al. Effects of Smoking on Inflammatory-Related Cytokine Levels in Human Serum. *Molecules*. 2022;27(12):3715. doi:https://doi.org/10.3390/molecules27123715
5. Alberts B, Johnson A, Lewis J, Raff M, Roberts K, Walter P. Blood Vessels and Endothelial Cells. *Molecular Biology of the Cell 4th Edition*. 2002;4. https://www.ncbi.nlm.nih.gov/books/NBK26848/#:~:text=Endothelial%20cells%20for m%20a%20single
6. Hahad O, Kuntic M, Kuntic I, Daiber A, Münzel T. Tobacco smoking and vascular biology and function: evidence from human studies. *Pflügers Archiv - European Journal of Physiology*. Published online March 24, 2023. doi:https://doi.org/10.1007/s00424-023-02805-z
7. Małgorzata Szkup, Jurczak A, Karakiewicz B, Artur Kotwas, Jacek Kopeć, Elżbieta Grochans. Influence of cigarette smoking on hormone and lipid metabolism in women in late reproductive stage. 2018;Volume 13:109-115. doi:https://doi.org/10.2147/cia.s140487
8. *TYPES of TOBACCO PRODUCTS*. https://portal.ct.gov/-/media/Departments-and-Agencies/DPH/dph/hems/tobacco/tobaccoproductspdf.pdf
9. Hartmann-Boyce J, Lindson N, Butler AR, et al. Electronic cigarettes for smoking cessation. *Cochrane Database of Systematic Reviews*. 2022;(11):CD010216. doi:10.1002/14651858.CD010216.pub7
10. 9 of the Worst Diseases You Can Get from Secondhand Smoke | State of Tobacco Control. www.lung.org. https://www.lung.org/research/sotc/by-the-numbers/9-diseases-secondhand-smoke
11. Miech R, Schulenberg J, Johnston L, Bachman J, O'Malley P, Patrick M. *Monitoring the Future National Adolescent Drug Trends in 2017: Findings Released*. Ann Arbor, MI: Institute for Social Research, The University of Michigan; 2017. https://monitoringthefuture.org/wp-content/uploads/2021/02/17drugpr.pdf Accessed January 2, 2018.
12. NIDA. How many adolescents use tobacco?. National Institute on Drug Abuse website. https://nida.nih.gov/publications/research-reports/tobacco-nicotine-e-

cigarettes/how-many-adolescents-use-tobacco. January 11, 2023 Accessed May 6, 2024.

13. Rahman MA, Hann N, Wilson A, Mnatzaganian G, Worrall-Carter L. E-Cigarettes and Smoking Cessation: Evidence from a Systematic Review and Meta-Analysis. PLoS ONE. 2015;10(3):e0122544. doi:10.1371/journal.pone.0122544

14. Jacobs M, Alonso AM, Sherin KM, et al. Policies to restrict secondhand smoke exposure: American College of Preventive Medicine Position Statement. *Am J Prev Med*. 2013;45(3):360-367. doi:10.1016/j.amepre.2013.05.007.

15. Prochaska JJ, Benowitz NL. The Past, Present, and Future of Nicotine Addiction Therapy. Annu Rev Med. 2016;67:467-86. doi: 10.1146/annurev-med-111314-033712. Epub 2015 Aug 26. PMID: 26332005; PMCID: PMC5117107.

16. Kofman M, Dunton K, Senkewicz MB. *Implementation of tobacco cessation coverage under the Affordable Care Act: understanding how private health insurance policies cover tobacco cessation treatments.* Health Policy Inst., Georgetown Univ, Washington, DC: 2012.

17. Raja M, Saha S, Mohd S, Narang R, Reddy LV, Kumari M. Cognitive Behavioural Therapy versus Basic Health Education for Tobacco Cessation among Tobacco Users: A Randomized Clinical Trail. *J Clin Diagn Res*. 2014;8(4):ZC47-ZC49. doi:10.7860/JCDR/2014/8015.4279

18. Lindson-Hawley N, Thompson TP, Begh R. Motivational interviewing for smoking cessation. *Cochrane Database Syst Rev*. 2015;(3):CD006936. Published 2015 Mar 2. doi:10.1002/14651858.CD006936.pub3

19. de Souza ICW, de Barros VV, Gomide HP, et al. Mindfulness-based interventions for the treatment of smoking: a systematic literature review. *J Altern Complement Med N Y N*. 2015;21(3):129-140. doi:10.1089/acm.2013.0471

20. Benowitz NL, Gourlay SG. Cardiovascular Toxicity of Nicotine: Implications for Nicotine Replacement Therapy 11All editorial decisions for this article, including selection of referees, were made by a Guest Editor. This policy applies to all articles with authors from the University of California San Francisco. *Journal of the American College of Cardiology*. 1997;29(7):1422-1431. doi:https://doi.org/10.1016/s0735-1097(97)00079-x

21. Carpenter MJ, Jardin BF, Burris JL, et al. Clinical strategies to enhance the efficacy of nicotine replacement therapy for smoking cessation: a review of the literature. *Drugs*. 2013;73(5):407-426. doi:10.1007/s40265-013-0038-y

22. Schnoll RA, Goelz PM, Veluz-Wilkins A, et al. Long-term nicotine replacement therapy: a randomized clinical trial. *JAMA Intern Med*. 2015;175(4):504-511. doi:10.1001/jamainternmed.2014.8313

23. Aubin H-J, Luquiens A, Berlin I. Pharmacotherapy for smoking cessation: pharmacological principles and clinical practice. *Br J Clin Pharmacol*. 2014;77(2):324-336. doi:10.1111/bcp.12116

24. Kaduri P, Voci S, Zawertailo L, Chaiton M, McKenzie K, Selby P. Real-world effectiveness of varenicline versus nicotine replacement therapy in patients with and without psychiatric disorders. *J Addict Med*. 2015;9(3):169-176. doi:10.1097/ADM.0000000000000111

25. Chang P-H, Chiang C-H, Ho W-C, Wu P-Z, Tsai J-S, Guo F-R. Combination therapy of varenicline with nicotine replacement therapy is better than varenicline alone: a systematic review and meta-analysis of randomized controlled trials. *BMC Public Health*. 2015;15:689. doi:10.1186/s12889-015-2055-0

26. Bellamoli E, Manganotti P, Schwartz RP, Rimondo C, Gomma M, Serpelloni G. rTMS in the treatment of drug addiction: an update about human studies. *Behav Neurol*. 2014;2014:815215. doi:10.1155/2014/815215

27. Haines-Saah RJ, Kelly MT, Oliffe JL, Bottorff JL. Picture Me Smokefree: a qualitative study using social media and digital photography to engage young adults in tobacco reduction and cessation. *J Med Internet Res*. 2015;17(1):e27. doi:10.2196/jmir.4061.

28. Ramo DE, Thrul J, Delucchi KL, Ling PM, Hall SM, Prochaska JJ. The Tobacco Status Project (TSP): Study protocol for a randomized controlled trial of a Facebook smoking cessation intervention for young adults. *BMC Public Health*. 2015;15:897. doi:10.1186/s12889-015-2217-0

29. Sally Dunlop, James Kite, Anne C. Grunseit, Chris Rissel, Donna A. Perez, Anita Dessaix, Trish Cotter, Adrian Bauman, Jane Young, David Currow, Out of Sight and Out of Mind? Evaluating the Impact of Point-of-Sale Tobacco Display Bans on Smoking-Related Beliefs and Behaviors in a Sample of Australian Adolescents and Young Adults, *Nicotine & Tobacco Research*, Volume 17, Issue 7, July 2015, Pages 761–768, https://doi.org/10.1093/ntr/ntu180

30. Danielsson A-K, Eriksson A-K, Allebeck P. Technology-based support via telephone or web: a systematic review of the effects on smoking, alcohol use and gambling. *Addict Behav*. 2014;39(12):1846-1868. doi:10.1016/j.addbeh.2014.06.007

31. Leung LWS, Davies GA. Smoking Cessation Strategies in Pregnancy. *J Obstet Gynecol Can JOGC*. 2015;37(9):791-797. doi:10.1016/S1701-2163(15)30149-3.

32. Tappin D, Bauld L, Purves D, et al. Financial incentives for smoking cessation in pregnancy: randomized controlled trial. *BMJ*. 2015;350:h134.

Hypertension: "The Silent Killer"
By: Priya Patel MD, Jonathan Kahan MD

What you need to know

1. High blood pressure, defined as a blood pressure of >130/80 mmHg is called the "silent killer" as it is highly prevalent (1 in 3 people worldwide) and is a major risk factor for heart attacks, strokes, kidney disease and death.
2. Goal blood pressure should be <130/80 mmHg for most people. Measuring blood pressure is tricky and there are strict steps to follow to check.
3. Treating blood pressure works! We have large, very well-done trials showing the enormous benefits of having normal blood pressures
4. Lifestyle changes, such as diet, weight loss and exercise work as well as medications and are the mainstay of treatment initially for everyone
5. For those who cannot achieve blood pressure goals, we have good classes of medications to get to our goal.

What is high blood pressure?

- Blood pressure is the pressure of blood pushing against the walls of your arteries measured in millimeters of mercury (mmHg) as seen in the picture below. Arteries carry blood from your heart to other parts of your body. Your blood pressure normally rises and falls throughout the day. The top number of blood pressure is when the heart squeezes (systolic blood pressure) and the bottom number is when the heart relaxes (diastolic blood pressure). High blood pressure is blood pressure higher than normal and if persistently elevated may result in the diagnosis of hypertension (1).

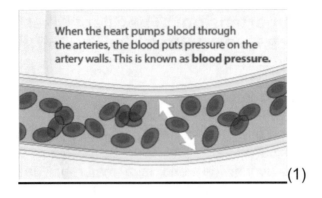

When the heart pumps blood through the arteries, the blood puts pressure on the artery walls. This is known as **blood pressure.**

(1)

How do we define high blood pressure?

- As per the American Heart Association (AHA) guidelines, hypertension is diagnosed when systolic blood pressure (SBP) in the office or clinic is ≥140 mm Hg and/or their diastolic blood pressure (DBP) is ≥90 mm Hg following repeated examination (2). Usually 2–3 office visits at 1–4-week intervals (depending on the BP level) are required to confirm the diagnosis of hypertension. The diagnosis might be made on a single visit, if BP is ≥180/110 mm Hg and there is evidence of cardiovascular disease (CVD) (3).

Blood Pressure Categories

American Heart Association.

BLOOD PRESSURE CATEGORY	SYSTOLIC mm Hg (upper number)		DIASTOLIC mm Hg (lower number)
NORMAL	LESS THAN 120	and	LESS THAN 80
ELEVATED	120-129	and	LESS THAN 80
HIGH BLOOD PRESSURE (HYPERTENSION) STAGE 1	130-139	or	80-89
HIGH BLOOD PRESSURE (HYPERTENSION) STAGE 2	140 OR HIGHER	or	90 OR HIGHER
HYPERTENSIVE CRISIS (consult your doctor immediately)	HIGHER THAN 180	and/or	HIGHER THAN 120

(3)

How common is high blood pressure?

- In 2021, hypertension was a primary contributing cause of 691,095 deaths in the United States and affects one out of every three people globally!
- Nearly half of adults have hypertension (48.1%, 119.9 million). About 1 in 4 adults with hypertension have their hypertension under control (22.5%, 27.0 million).
- High blood pressure costs the United States about $131 billion each year, averaged over 12 years from 2003 to 2014. (4)

US adults with hypertension[b] 48.1% (119.9 million)		
Recommended intervention type — Lifestyle modifications only 20.9% (25.0 million)	Lifestyle modifications plus medication 79.1% (94.9 million)	
Blood pressure control status[c] — Uncontrolled 77.5% (92.9 million)		Controlled 22.5% (27.0 million)

Why should I care about high blood pressure?

- Having prolonged untreated blood pressure has many consequences, one of which is a stroke, either a hemorrhagic stroke (bleed in the brain) or ischemic stroke where a clot breaks off and stops blood flow to the brain. Other adverse outcomes include vision loss by damaging blood vessels in the eyes.

- It can also cause a heart attack by causing more stress on the heart causing a supply-demand mismatch and breaking off of plaque leading to a blockage. Untreated high blood pressure can also lead to heart failure, which is a scary term but over time, high blood pressure causes thickening of the left ventricle, the main pumping chamber of the heart. Eventually, the left ventricle becomes thin, dilated and does not pump well leading to its own set of complications.

- High blood pressure also affects your kidneys and their function by causing damage to the small blood vessels in the kidney and causing leaking of important proteins and eventually leading to kidney failure and dialysis. People can also experience sexual dysfunction such as erectile dysfunction.

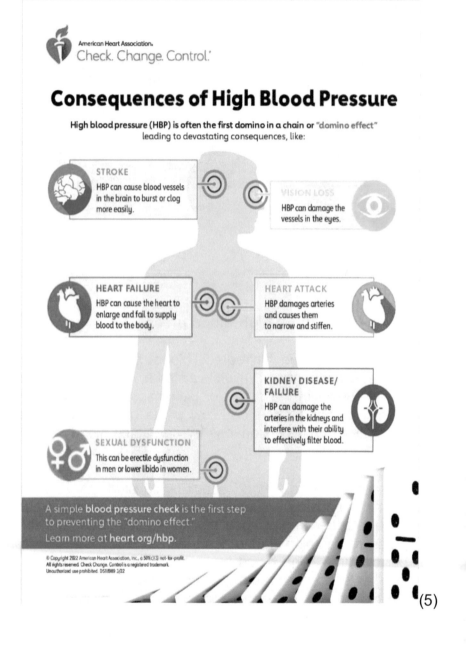

(5)

How do I check my blood pressure?

- When measuring blood pressure, ideally you should not have exercised, smoked, or had caffeine in the last 30 minutes.
- Don't eat or drink anything 30 minutes before you take your blood pressure.
- Empty your bladder before checking your blood pressure.
- Sit in a comfortable chair with your back supported for at least 5 minutes before your reading.
- Put both feet flat on the ground and keep your legs uncrossed.
- Rest your arm with the cuff on a table at chest height.
- Make sure the blood pressure cuff is snug but not too tight. The cuff should be against your bare skin, not over clothing.
- Do not talk while your blood pressure is being measured (2).
- The best brand for home blood pressure cuff is Omron, but it can still be accurate 15% of the time. It is important to correlate home blood pressure cuff with blood pressure cuff at your doctor's office.

What symptoms can I experience with high blood pressure?

Most individuals are asymptomatic (which is why high blood pressure is called the silent killer), other symptoms that you can experience include (7):
- Headaches
- Blurred vision
- Nocturia (urinating at night)
- Hematuria (blood in the urine)
- Dizziness
- Chest pain
- Shortness of breath
- Palpitations

What are the risk factors for high blood pressure?

Risk factors can be broken down into modifiable and relatively fixed risk factors (2):

Modifiable risk factors include:

29

- Diabetes mellitus
- Obesity
- Dyslipidemia/hypercholesterolemia
- Physical inactivity
- Obstructive sleep apnea
- Unhealthy diet

Relatively fixed risk factors include:
- Chronic kidney disease
- Genetics/family history
- Age

Why do people have high blood pressure?

- The short answer is we do not have just one cause, but rather multiple different etiologies such as genetics, dietary salt intake, obesity, sedentary lifestyle, increased alcohol intake, stress can all lead to high blood pressure (8).

- Obesity-related hypertension is caused by a complex neuro-hormonal cascade in the body that activates pathways brain, kidneys and adipose tissue (fat cells) leading to hypertension. A similar process occurs with stress. Increased stress may be due to a job, a visit to the doctor's office, social/environmental or emotional stressors can increase release of vasoconstricting hormones that increase blood pressure (9).

What about salt?

- You will hear us talk incessantly about salt. Why does salt intake matter because salty things taste good, right? Well, this is true but salt causes the body to retain water which increases total blood volume resulting in increased blood pressure. So, you may be asking, what can I do? First, take the salt shaker off the table (our goal daily salt intake is less than 2.5 grams). Second, just having one glass of water before eating a satly meal (such as a restaurant) will help control your blood pressure by reducing the blood osmolarity (salt concentration relative to blood volume) from salt intake to reduce the spike in blood pressure (10). Fascinating, I know.

You still with me? Don't fall asleep because we have a bit more to talk about.

What are other causes of high blood pressure?

I won't bore you with the details but here are some other terms and causes of to be aware of:

- Primary or commonly referred to as essential hypertension is the most common cause of high blood pressure in the general population and the etiology is unknown but we do know that obesity, poor diet, high alcohol intake, increased salt intake can lead to essential hypertension. It typically begins in those over the age of 30, and often with a family history of hypertension (8).
- Secondary hypertension is related to a specific etiology and is often resistant to treatment. It can be sudden in onset or be labile and difficult to control especially in a person without family history. Some causes to be aware of are below (8,11):
  - Obstructive sleep apnea
  - Primary aldosteronism
  - Renal parenchymal disease like chronic kidney disease, polycystic kidney disease, glomerulonephritis
  - Renovascular disease like renal artery stenosis or fibromuscular dysplasia
  - Endocrine or hormonal dysregulation like Cushing's syndrome, hyperthyroidism/hypothyroidism, primary hyperparathyroidism, pheochromocytoma/paraganglioma
  - Vascular or blood vessel disorder like aortic coarctation or aortitis/vasculitis

How do I control my high blood pressure?

- Before we get in the how, we need to go over the blood pressure goals and when we start treating high blood pressure. When blood pressure remains over >140/>90, we start treating with medications (2).

- **The goal for basically everyone is to have a blood pressure of <130/<80 mmHg (2)**
- The higher the risk you are for heart attacks and strokes, the more important treating blood pressure becomes. The tradeoff are things like dizziness, passing out and kidney injury from low blood pressure.
- Women with hypertension who are pregnant or planning to get pregnant should be transitioned to labetalol, methyldopa, and nifedipine during pregnancy. Goal blood pressure is 140/90 as per American College of Gynecology guidelines (12).

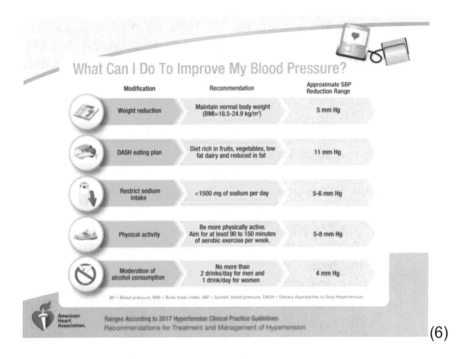

(6)

Now that we discussed what the treatment goal for blood pressure should be, let us talk about how to manage it.

- **Diet, weight loss and exercise are by far the best treatment for blood pressure.**
- The Dietary Approaches to Stop Hypertension (AKA DASH) diet which includes eating vegetables, fruits and whole grains including fat free or low-fat dairy products, fish, poultry, beans, nut and vegetable oils. Limit foods high in fatty meats and limit sugar sweetened beverages and sweets which can lead to about 11 mmHg drop in blood pressure. Sugar intake

increases stimulation of the sympathetic nervous system in the brain activating a neuro-hormonal cascade and causes vasoconstriction causing blood pressure to rise (13).

- Decreasing salt intake to less than 2.3 grams of salt per day can lead to an additional 5-6 mmHg decrease in blood pressure (14).
- Weight loss, ideally to lose about 1 kg of weight and expect about 1 mmHg decrease in blood pressure with every 1 kg reduction in body weight (2).

- Physical activity (see exercise section for a much more complete guide):
  - Aerobic activity about 90 to 150 minutes per week, target heart rate 65- 75% of your age (2)
  - Dynamic Resistance about 90 to 150 minutes per week, target heart rate 50-80% of your age (2)
  - Isometric Resistance to be done 4 times for 2 minutes, 1 minute rest between exercises. Do 30-40% maximum voluntary contraction, 3 sessions per week for 8-10 weeks. (2)

- Moderation of alcohol consumption, reduce to ≤ 2 drinks per week or cessation of alcohol use (2).

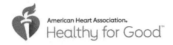

American Heart Association. Healthy for Good™

DID YOU KNOW?

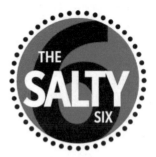

THE SALTY SIX

These six popular foods can add high levels of sodium to your diet.	As part of a healthy dietary pattern that emphasizes the intake of vegetables, fruits, nuts, whole grains, lean vegetable or animal protein, and fish and minimizes the intake of trans fats, red meat and processed red meats, refined carbohydrates, and sugary drinks, the American Heart Association recommends 2,300 milligrams (mgs) or less a day of sodium.*

Daily suggested sodium referenced below is based on 2,300 mgs/day recommendation:

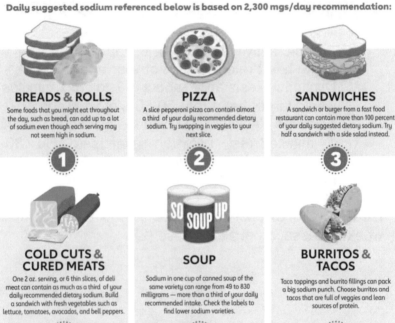

BREADS & ROLLS
Some foods that you might eat throughout the day, such as bread, can add up to a lot of sodium even though each serving may not seem high in sodium.

1

PIZZA
A slice pepperoni pizza can contain almost a third of your daily recommended dietary sodium. Try swapping in veggies to your next slice.

2

SANDWICHES
A sandwich or burger from a fast food restaurant can contain more than 100 percent of your daily suggested dietary sodium. Try half a sandwich with a side salad instead.

3

COLD CUTS & CURED MEATS
One 2 oz. serving, or 6 thin slices, of deli meat can contain as much as a third of your daily recommended dietary sodium. Build a sandwich with fresh vegetables such as lettuce, tomatoes, avocados, and bell peppers.

4

SOUP
Sodium in one cup of canned soup of the same variety can range from 49 to 830 milligrams — more than a third of your daily recommended intake. Check the labels to find lower sodium varieties.

5

BURRITOS & TACOS
Taco toppings and burrito fillings can pack a big sodium punch. Choose burritos and tacos that are full of veggies and lean sources of protein.

6

Compare labels whenever possible and choose options with the lower amounts of added sugars, sodium and saturated fat and no trans fat and look out for the Heart-Check mark, a simple tool to help you eat smart. When you see it, you can be confident that a product aligns with the American Heart Association's recommendations for an overall healthy eating pattern, including sodium.

*Also, remember serving size makes a difference. Eating double the serving size means you are eating double the sodium. 1,500 mg/d for those who are sensitive to sodium and /or at high risk for hypertension.

© Copyright 2020 American Heart Association, Inc., a 501(c)(3) not-for-profit. All rights reserved. Unauthorized use prohibited. DS15225 2/20

(15)

I have done all the changes, yet lifestyle isn't enough!
When lifestyle isn't enough, we give you a boost with medications and we have multiple medications in our armament to choose from

as the first line. The class of medications that are first line are the calcium channel blockers, the thiazide diuretics and the angiotensin receptor blockers/angiotensin converting enzymes. Remember our goal is <130/80 mmHg most days.

- First line medications for blood pressure management includes thiazide and thiazide like diuretics such as chlorthalidone, hydrochlorothiazide, metolazone or indapamide. These medications are water pills and will make you urinate frequently in order to reduce blood volume. Common side effects include electrolyte abnormalities, dizziness, lightheadedness, and dehydration (16).
- Calcium channel blockers like amlodipine, nifedipine, felodipine are vasodilators and cause dilation of blood vessels and decrease blood pressure. These medications provide a steady control of blood pressure throughout the day without spikes. Common side effects lower extremity swelling (most common), headache and constipation (16).
- ACE inhibitors like enalapril, lisinopril and angiotensin receptor blocker (ARB) like Valsartan, Losartan, Olmesartan. These medications dilate blood vessels in the kidneys to reduce blood pressure. This group of medications are often first line in patients with diabetes mellitus, chronic kidney disease, heart failure. Common side effects include cough (more with ACE inhibitors), elevation in renal function (temporarily), hyperkalemia (elevated blood potassium level), angioedema (facial swelling). After starting these medications, repeat labs are done within 1-2 weeks to check renal function and potassium levels (16).
- Beta blockers like atenolol, metoprolol, carvedilol or labetalol can be used for blood pressure but often not the first choice (because they are weaker) unless some has a history of heart attack, heart failure or tachycardia (fast heart rate). Common side effects include fatigue, slow heart rate and sexual dysfunction (16). Other blood pressure medications that can be used include loop diuretics like furosemide or torsemide.
- Potassium sparing diuretics like eplerenone or spironolactone can be used in resistant hypertension cases or in patients with heart failure.
- Less common medications include minoxidil, clonidine and alpha blockers like terazosin or prazosin.

35

Medication category	Examples	Common side effects
ACE inhibitors	Lisinopril, captopril, enalapril	Dry cough, swelling of face and lips, high potassium, decreased GFR
Angiotensin receptor blockers (ARB)	Losartan, valsartan	High potassium, decreased GFR
Calcium channel blocker	Amlodipine, nifedipine	Leg edema, headache, constipation
Beta blockers	Carvedilol, metoprolol, atenolol	Dizziness, slow heart rate, tiredness, sexual dysfunction
Thiazide diuretics	Hydrochlorothiazide, chlorthalidone	Low potassium, weakness, leg cramps, gout
Alpha blockers	Prazosin, doxazosin	Fast heart rate, low blood pressure, dizziness, weakness

References:

1.Centers for Disease Control and Prevention. About high blood pressure (hypertension). Centers for Disease Control and Prevention. Published May 18, 2021. https://www.cdc.gov/bloodpressure/about.htm
2. Whelton PK, Carey RM, Aronow WS, et al. 2017 ACC/AHA/AAPA/ABC/ACPM/AGS/APhA/ASH/ASPC/NMA/PCNA Guideline for the Prevention, Detection, Evaluation, and Management of High Blood Pressure in Adults: A Report of the American College of Cardiology/American Heart Association Task Force on Clinical Practice Guidelines. Hypertension. 2018;71(6). doi:https://doi.org/10.1161/hyp.0000000000000065
3. American Heart Association. Understanding Blood Pressure Readings. American Heart Association. Published May 30, 2023. https://www.heart.org/en/health-topics/high-blood-pressure/understanding-blood-pressure-readings
4. Centers for Disease Control and Prevention. Hypertension Prevalence in the U.S. | Million Hearts®. Centers for Disease Control and Prevention. Published May 12, 2023. https://millionhearts.hhs.gov/data-reports/hypertension-prevalence.html
5. Consequences of High Blood Pressure. https://www.heart.org/-/media/Files/Health-Topics/High-Blood-Pressure/Consequences-of-High-Blood-Pressure-infographic.pdf
6. What Can I Do To Improve My High Blood Pressure? targetbp.org. Accessed April 12, 2024. https://targetbp.org/tools_downloads/what-can-i-do-to-improve-my-blood-pressure/
7. World Health Organization. Hypertension. World Health Organization. Published 2023. https://www.who.int/news-room/fact-sheets/detail/hypertension
8. Carretero OA, Oparil S. Essential hypertension. Part I: definition and etiology. Circulation. 2000;101(3):329-335. doi:https://doi.org/10.1161/01.cir.101.3.329
9. Shariq OA, McKenzie TJ. Obesity-related hypertension: a review of pathophysiology, management, and the role of metabolic surgery. Gland Surgery. 2020;9(1):80-93. doi:https://doi.org/10.21037/gs.2019.12.03

10. Kanbay M, Aslan G, Afsar B, et al. Acute effects of salt on blood pressure are mediated by serum osmolality. *The Journal of Clinical Hypertension*. 2018;20(10):1447-1454. doi:https://doi.org/10.1111/jch.13374

11. Chapter 13. Secondary hypertension. *Hypertension Research*. 2014;37(4):349-361. doi:https://doi.org/10.1038/hr.2014.16

12. Clinical Guidance for the Integration of the Findings of the Chronic Hypertension and Pregnancy (CHAP) Study. www.acog.org. https://www.acog.org/clinical/clinical-guidance/practice-advisory/articles/2022/04/clinical-guidance-for-the-integration-of-the-findings-of-the-chronic-hypertension-and-pregnancy-chap-study#:~:text=Based%20on%20these%20findings%2C%20ACOG

13. Mansoori S, Kushner N, Suminski RR, Farquhar WB, Chai SC. Added Sugar Intake is Associated with Blood Pressure in Older Females. *Nutrients*. 2019;11(9):2060. doi:https://doi.org/10.3390/nu11092060

14. Sacks FM, Svetkey LP, Vollmer WM, et al. Effects on blood pressure of reduced dietary sodium and the Dietary Approaches to Stop Hypertension (DASH) diet. DASH-Sodium Collaborative Research Group. *The New England journal of medicine*. 2001;344(1):3-10. doi:https://doi.org/10.1056/NEJM200101043440101

15. Northwest Arkansas LifestyleRX. www.heart.org. Accessed April 12, 2024. https://www.heart.org/en/affiliates/nwalifestylerx

16. Khalil H, Zeltser R. Antihypertensive Medications. PubMed. Published May 8, 2023. https://www.ncbi.nlm.nih.gov/books/NBK554579/

Cholesterol/Lipids
By: Mohamed Hamed MD, Eric Lieberman MD, Jonathan Kahan MD

What you need to know:

1. Lipids include both cholesterol and triglycerides, which are molecules of fat necessary for life. However, when our lipids are too high, they can cause plaque to develop in the arteries of our body, leading to most cardiovascular diseases.
2. This is a slow process, with buildup of plaque beginning in childhood and progressing over decades. There needs to be a combination of cholesterol plaque ("wood") and inflammation ("sparks") from the immune system in order to create unstable plaques that rupture ("fire"), leading to heart attacks and strokes.
3. The standard lipid profile blood test has many pitfalls and moving to testing for the protein carriers of lipids, such as Apolipoproteins B and E, as well as the most atherogenic lipoprotein "little" a, are beneficial and much more relevant in terms of cardiovascular outcomes.
4. While smoking, diet, and lifestyle can have profound effects on cholesterol, there is a larger genetic component here than other sections of the book. Hints to a genetic cause are seen in the lipid profile and can then be confirmed by genetic analysis. Because of this, pharmacotherapy here is more important as patient's may not be able to change their lipid profiles significantly.

What are lipids? What is cholesterol? What are triglycerides?

Lipids include both cholesterol and triglyceride and are non-soluble (does not dissolve in water) molecules that are transported by lipoproteins (proteins which are soluble, and therefore can be carried by blood which is mainly water) [1,2,3]. Triglycerides (TG) are made up of three (3) fatty acid molecules attached to a glycerol backbone. These fatty acids are further classified into monounsaturated (aka omega 9), polyunsaturated (omega 3,6), saturated, or trans fats. Triglycerides (TG) outweigh cholesterol 10-

100x in animal products. Plants do not contain cholesterol but have triglycerides [4,5].

Lipids are essential for your health, but too much of certain kinds of cholesterol/triglycerides can increase the risk of cardiovascular disease (this is called hyperlipidemia). Note that there really isn't "bad" and "good" cholesterol as you will see below.

What does cholesterol do in the body? What do triglycerides do in the body?

Cholesterol is used for cell structure and function (especially cell membrane formation), in energy production, steroid hormones synthesis, bile acid production, and storage and transport of fat-soluble vitamins (Vitamins A, D, E and K) [6,7].

Triglycerides are used mainly for energy, both as a source and for storage, as well as insulation/protection in the form of adipose/fat cells. They are also part of cell membranes [8].

What is a lipoprotein?

Lipoproteins are complex molecular structures composed of fats and proteins. They are responsible for transporting lipids to various organs. Think of a lipoprotein as a spherical cage that holds within it a liquid core of lipids. They are necessary because lipids are insoluble (think oil in water) and so they transport lipids around the body [9,10]. We are concerned with 4 of them:

1. Apolipoprotein A1: the spherical protein cage that contains HDL (high density lipids).
2. Apolipoprotein B (ApoB): the spherical protein cage that contains VLDL (very low-density lipids), IDL (intermediate density lipids) and LDL (low density lipids).
3. Lipoprotein "little" a (Lp(a)): the exact same as a small LDL/ApoB just with an extra protein tail.
4. Apolipoprotein E: the protein cage critical to transporting lipids and heavy metals across the blood brain barrier (both ways) and involved in neuron growth and repair.

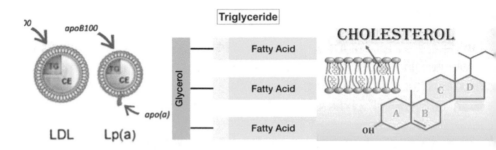

Glavinovic T, Thanassoulis G, de Graaf J, Couture P, Hegele RA, Sniderman AD. Physiological Bases for the Superiority of Apolipoprotein B Over Low-Density Lipoprotein Cholesterol and Non–High-Density Lipoprotein Cholesterol as a Marker of Cardiovascular Risk. *Journal of the American Heart Association.* 2022;11(20). doi:https://doi.org/10.1161/jaha.122.025858

Study Mind. Lipids and Triglycerides (A-level Biology). Study Mind. https://studymind.co.uk/notes/lipids-and-triglycerides/

Figure: Structures of 3 different molecules. The first on the left is an apoB protein holding a liquid center of cholesterols (CE) and triglycerides (TG). The liquid cholesterol center is like oil, which cannot dissolve in water. The apoB protein acts like a spiral cage which can dissolve in water (i.e. blood) and therefore move around the body, dropping off its liquid cargo at various sites. ApoB is the common carrier protein. The main difference between Lp(a) and ApoB is that it has lost most of its triglyceride cargo and has an extra tail. Triglycerides are 3 fatty acids connected to glycero (middle pic). Cholesterol is structured as four linked hydrocarbon rings (right pic) [9-15].

How do we go from consuming cholesterol/triglycerides to plaque buildup in the arteries of our hearts/organs (aka atherosclerosis)?

Note: See appendix for the full picture. It is very complicated, however understanding it will allow you to see how all the lipids relate to cardiovascular disease. A good analogy is this: cholesterol is the "wood" and inflammation is the "sparks" that create the fire of plaque rupture. Note inflammation is chronic here and comes from metabolic dysfunction +/- smoke inhalation. Below is a "brief" summary:

When we consume lipids (cholesterol and TG) they are broken down in our stomach and get absorbed into our bloodstream inside of a protein cage called a chylomicron via the small intestines. On the way to the liver the chylomicron drops off TG to our muscles for energy/storage and to our fat cells for storage. In the liver, the remaining cholesterol/TG can be either made into bile acids to go back to the GI tract for cholesterol absorption, be packaged in an apoB cage to become VLDL or an apoA1 cage to become HDL. VLDL goes to the muscles/fat cells to drop off even more cholesterol/TG, becoming LDL, while HDL goes to tissues and brings cholesterol/TG back to the liver. Lp(a), which is made in the liver, is exactly the same as a small LDL just with a protein tail [16,17].

VLDL, LDL and Lp(a) particles can get stuck in the lining of the arteries of organs. They then become oxidized by free radicals, smoke, reactive oxygen species etc which causes immune cells to attack them (creating a foam cell), leading to inflammation and plaque formation (aka atherosclerosis). Fat cells/metabolic dysfunction creates cytokines (messenger molecules) that can speed up this process. Plaques start off as small but with a thin cap (see pic below), which is also called a vulnerable plaque. When this cap breaks, the liquid, inflammatory center is exposed to the bloodstream where the body attacks it, and it becomes much larger very rapidly. This plaque rupture happens repeatedly and dynamically until 100% blockage is created. This is how heart attacks, strokes, congestive heart failure and death from cardiovascular disease occur. It is usually a sudden process at the end, however it starts when we are approximately 8 years old! [16-20] Note: See obesity chapter for how cholesterol/TG dropped off in muscle and other organs leads to metabolic dysfunction.

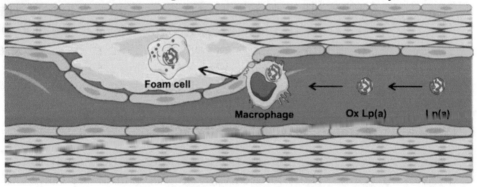

Ugovšek S, Šebeštjen M. Lipoprotein(a)—The Crossroads of Atherosclerosis, Atherothrombosis and Inflammation. *Biomolecules.* 2022; 12(1):26. https://doi.org/10.3390/biom12010026

Where does Cholesterol come from? Where do triglycerides come from?

1. **Endogenous:** Cholesterol and triglycerides are produced within the body (primarily the liver) and are highly affected by genetics and environmental factors. Note 70-80% of cholesterol comes from endogenous production [21,22]. This is why pharmacologic intervention may be of use here.

2. **Dietary:** comes through consumption of foods, especially animal-derived foods. The main sources are meat, eggs, cheese, and dairy products. The relationship between ingestion of dietary cholesterol and cholesterol in blood is weak at best. Note eggs have 200 mg of cholesterol each and is what is studied most (because they are easy to count and standardize). For example, the PURE trial showed that higher egg intake [[>7 eggs/week vs, none] was not associated with any changes in cholesterol/blood lipids or any CVD outcomes. Similar results were found in ONTARGET and TRANSCEND trails (taken together >175,000 patients). Importantly, while the CHNS trial showed a decrease in all-cause mortality from eggs; red meat, pork, cheese and butter did not have the same results, which may relate more to other properties in eggs vs. meat. Note that following a low sugar diet can lead to a decrease in triglyceride levels [21,23-26].

   a. Excess carbohydrates specifically added sugars like glucose and fructose lead to preferential creation of triglycerides in the liver, which is sent to muscle cells and fat cells causing dysfunction (see obesity chapter).

What are the different types of fatty acids?

Remember that a triglyceride is just 3 fatty acids attached to a glycerol backbone. They can be in any combination of the fatty acids below:

1. Monounsaturated fats (MUFAs): Monounsaturated fats (olive oil, canola oil, peanut oil) have one double bond between

carbon atoms and stay liquid at room temperature. These are also called Omega-9s (oleic acid is the common omega-9 in olive oil and 70% of the fats in avocado). Consuming monounsaturated fats increase HDL cholesterol and lower LDL cholesterol.

2. Polyunsaturated fats (PUFAs): Have more than one double bond and stay liquid at room temperature (soybean oil, corn oil, nuts, seeds, fatty fish). PUFAs are broken down into Omega-3s (fatty fish, walnuts, chia, flax) and Omega-6s (soy, corn, sunflower, safflower oils). Note: these types of triglycerides are most vulnerable to oxidation outside the body (think rancid fish oil), leading to all the problems of oxidized lipids that are stuck in arteries of the body.

3. Trans fat: (think margarine, puff pastry, olive oil when it's burnt): also unsaturated but have a different configuration making them solid at room temperature. Trans fats raise LDL levels, create reactive oxygen species, promote inflammation and plaque formation. These fats have largely been banned in North America.

4. Saturated fats, which have no double bonds between molecules and stay solid at room temperature (think butter, cheese, red meats). Consuming saturated fats does raise low -density lipoprotein (LDL) cholesterol by increasing apolipoprotein B production and decreasing the LDL receptor activity in the liver. However, consuming saturated fats also raises high density lipoprotein (HDL) and therefore the total cholesterol to HDL ratio (a marker for CVD) remains the same. Note eating a high saturated fat diet has not translated to improved CVD outcomes in large studies such as the Minnesota Heart Study when compared to vegetable oil. [27-30]

What evidence Is there that elevated cholesterol and triglycerides lead to CVD?

There are multiple large trials that have shown that elevated cholesterol and triglycerides lead to CVD. On the cholesterol side the Framingham Heart Study (one of the most famous cardiovascular studies) showed strong correlation between LDL cholesterol and CVD. Similarly on the TG side, the Copenhagen City Heart Study showed fasting TG were independently associated with risk of heart attacks and ischemic heart disease, independent of age, smoking etc. [31-33]

How do we measure lipids?

The most common method used to measure lipid levels is the lipid profile.

What is lipid profile?

The lipid profile includes total cholesterol, high-density lipoprotein (HDL)-cholesterol, triglycerides (TGs) and low-density lipoprotein (LDL)-cholesterol (LDL-C). It is used as an important method for the risk assessment for cardiovascular disease.

VLDL and LDL-C have traditionally been calculated using the **Friedewald equation,** not through direct measurement. VLDL is calculated by TG/5 and LDL is calculated by Total cholesterol - HDL - VLDL [34].

What are the Pitfalls of these calculations?

This equation is not valid when the **Triglyceride** level is ≥400 mg/dL or <100 mg/dL. Also, TG varies with state of fasting, recent meals, recent alcohol use and metabolic conditions such as DM. You can measure LDL directly with an additional blood test order. Studies suggest repeating the LDL by direct assay techniques in patients with triglyceride >200 mg/dL or when LDL<70 or >130 mg/dL [34-36].

Are there limitations for direct LDL-C assays?

So, what is the problem with measuring LDL directly? There are no standard methods to directly measure LDL-C. There are multiple assays to direct LDL-C produced from different manufacturers and different labs use different assays which can show inaccurate results.

It is more expensive for direct LDL-C measurement as it needs additional reagents and labor compared with the calculated LDL-C method. You may have also heard about measuring the different densities of LDL, with small dense LDL being more atherogenic. However, the same exact problems persist, in that different labs use different magnets to measure the density of LDL, and there are no standards. Furthermore, it doesn't include the most atherogenic particle which is Lp(a) [36-38].

What is the most accurate way of measuring "bad cholesterol" and cardiac risk?

Apo B is the protein on all VLDL, IDL, LDL particles and Lp(a) can be measured directly. These labs are unrelated to the baseline state of the patient and are uniform among all laboratories. Elevated levels of apo B are associated with increased risk of cardiovascular disease. There is substantial evidence that apoB levels measure the atherogenic risk better than LDL or non-HDL cholesterol. In addition, only ApoB particles [and Lp(a)] can enter the artery wall and create atherosclerosis [39-41].

apoB lipoproteins

Glavinovic T, Thanassoulis G, de Graaf J, Couture P, Hegele RA, Sniderman AD. Physiological Bases for the Superiority of Apolipoprotein B Over Low-Density Lipoprotein Cholesterol and Non–High-Density Lipoprotein Cholesterol as a Marker of Cardiovascular Risk. *Journal of the American Heart Association*. 2022;11(20). doi:https://doi.org/10.1161/jaha.122.025858

Approximately half of all patients with recurrent heart attacks have normal cholesterol levels on standard lipid profiles, and despite having achieved the recommended LDL, these patients are still at high risk of cardiovascular-related events. Because there is a 1:1 relationship between an apoB molecule and an LDL core, it always correlates to risk of CVD. If there are numerous apoB molecules but each one carries normal LDL amounts, then the LDL measurement in blood will be normal, despite elevated risk. Conversely, large LDL cores can lead to falsely elevated LDL levels, which exaggerate risk, despite normal apoB levels. This occurs in 7% of diabetic patients and 15% of patients with metabolic syndrome have normal apoB with elevated LDL. These patients do not develop cardiovascular disease and do not need cholesterol lowering therapy [39-43]. Apo B level more than 130 mg/dl is considered elevated risk for cardiovascular disease [44].

What elevates ApoB?

1. Diet: diet high in saturated fats and trans fats can increase the production and secretion of apoB-containing lipoproteins.
2. Obesity: Visceral fat (see obesity section) can secrete various hormones and cytokines that influence lipid metabolism and increase the levels of apoB-containing lipoproteins.
3. Physical inactivity: sedentary lifestyle and lack of regular exercise. Exercise increases metabolic demand from muscles, increasing free fatty acid and TG use. Additionally, it raises HDL levels (think revving up the system), enhances LDL receptor activity in the liver to suck back cholesterol particles and reduces the metabolically active visceral fat.
4. Genetics: genetic factors which include mutations in genes involved in lipid metabolism. For example: familial hypercholesterolemia. Genetic factors are prominent in lipid disorders. Again, this is the one area where pharmacology will play a more prominent role.
5. Insulin resistance including conditions like metabolic syndrome and diabetes mellitus.
6. Liver diseases: The liver is the most important organ in lipid metabolism and impaired liver function can disrupt lipid metabolism leading to elevated levels of apoB.
7. Smoking: Tobacco smoking has been associated with dyslipidemia and increased levels of apoB-containing lipoproteins. [39-43]

What is Lipoprotein(a) [Lp (a) aka Lp "little" a]

Lp (a) is a type of lipoprotein particle composed of LDL cholesterol (in an apoB) and bound to apolipoprotein(a) (the tail). It can induce vascular inflammation, atherogenesis, calcification and thrombosis because it is the smallest cholesterol particle. Lp (a) levels are heavily determined by genetics. Patients with family history of elevated Lp(a) are at increased risk for cardiovascular disease and it may even cause aortic valve narrowing. It cannot be influenced by lifestyle factors like diet and exercise in the same way other particles are [38,45-47]. The optimal Lp(a) levels < 14 mg/dL. Patients with Lp (a) levels 14-30 mg/dL are considered at borderline risk, while patients with Lp (a) range of 31-50 mg/dL are at high risk. Lp (a) levels higher than 50 mg/dL confer the highest risk range for cardiovascular disease [46].

- The higher the level of Lp(a) the higher the risk of MACE (major adverse cardiac event)

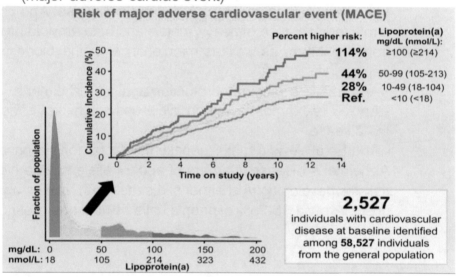

Martel J. Lp(a). Quatuor MD. Published July 24, 2023. Accessed May 1, 2024. https://quatuormd.ca/en/lpa/

N.B Statins and ezetimibe (Zetia) do not effectively lower Lp(a), in fact they may paradoxically increase its concentrations up to 30%. PSCK-9 inhibitors can decrease the levels by 30-40%. There are specific drugs targeting Lp (a) in development [48-50].

What is Apolipoprotein E (Apo E)?

Apo E is a protein involved in lipid metabolism and transport, especially in the blood brain barrier (a series of blood vessels that surround the brain, controlling what gets in/out). There are 3 major variants: apoE2, apoE3 and apoE4. A Blood test can determine allele status (E2E2, E2E3, E2E4, E3E3, E3E4, and E4E4) [51-53].

What does ApoE do?

- Cholesterol transport: It has a key role in the metabolism of lipoproteins and cholesterol transport. In addition, it has an important role in the removal of triglyceride-rich lipoproteins from the circulation.
- Alzheimer's disease: It has been implicated that apoE has a role in the pathogenesis of Alzheimer's disease. Apo E has a role for clearance of heavy metals and beta amyloid protein from the brain, as well as maintenance of the blood brain barrier.
  - Apo E2 allele provides protection against Alzheimer's.
  - Apo E3 is the most common allele and has neural effect on the disease
  - Apo E4 allele is a major genetic risk factor for the onset of Alzheimer's disease. Carriers of apo E4 allele have a higher risk for developing Alzheimer's disease with earlier age of onset. Around 15-25% of people have at least one allele copy [51-54].

APO-E and likelihood for development of Alzheimer's dementia

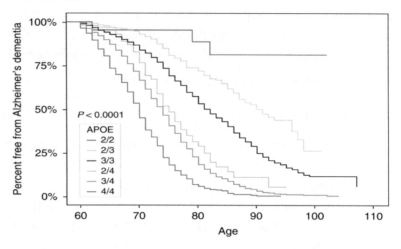

Reiman EM, Arboleda-Velasquez JF, Quiroz YT, et al. Exceptionally low likelihood of Alzheimer's dementia in APOE2 homozygotes from a 5,000-person neuropathological study. *Nature Communications.* 2020;11(1).doi:https://doi.org/10.1038/s41467-019-14279-8

- The apo E4 allele responds significantly to a low saturated fat diet (more so than pharmacologic intervention), resulting in lower apoB and triglycerides and a potential decreased risk of developing Alzheimer's dementia (evidence limited for this). It is controversial whether omega-3 has an effect. Overall, we recommend the aggressive lifestyle, diet and pharmacologic interventions in this book if you are diagnosed with an APOE-4 allele [54].

Wait, so I can inherit cholesterol issues?

Yes! There are a multitude of common inherited hyperlipidemia disorders called familial hyperlipidemias. We suspect a patient may have these if they have a personal or family history of early cardiovascular disease (defined as a CVD event in men before the age of 55 and women before the age of 65), abnormally high lipid levels despite diet and exercise (especially in children), and certain physical characteristics. Classically, familial hyperlipidemia with isolated high LDL responds extremely well to a low saturated fat diet (affects 1 in 250 people). Familial Hypertrigliceridemia may respond to omega 3 fatty acids or other lipid lowering therapies. The most common is familial combined hyperlipidemia which affects 1 in 50 people! It is one of the few cholesterol conditions that responds well to a combined low saturated fat and high omega 3 diets. The rest will require some combination of lifestyle and cholesterol lowering medication (see below). This class of cholesterol issues belies the importance of checking lipid profiles early! [55-57]

Ok ok, so what are the general goals of treatment for lipids?

Guidelines vary, however the generic answer is the lower the better. We have not found a patient who has "too low" cholesterol. Infants have a total cholesterol of around 10-20 mg/dL to put things in perspective. Also remember that plaques begin to form when a person is around 8 years old, so the younger the better to start treatment also is vital [20,58].

Who currently gets treatment for Cholesterol?

The most commonly used guidelines are the **US Preventive Services Task Force** (USPTF) guidelines.

Current USPTF guidelines:

1. Adults who are age 40-75 with at least one CVD risk factor (smoking, HTN etc)

2. ASCVD risk 7.5% (consider prevention), >10% recommend prevention

3. Diabetics

4. LDL > 190 mg/dL

Note: Currently it is not recommended to start statin therapy in patients aged 76 or older for primary prevention by the USPTF [59,60]

What is ASCVD?

ASCVD (Atherosclerotic cardiovascular disease) is a risk calculator using various parameters to gauge a person's 10-year risk of having a heart attack or stroke [61]. It is used heavily for determining a patient's risk however several problems come up which in our opinion limits its use.

App intended for primary prevention patients (without ASCVD) who have LDL-C < 190 mg/dL (4.921 mmol/L)

Current Age ❶ *   Sex *   Race *
[   ] | Male | Female | | White | African American | Other |
Age must be between 40-79

Systolic Blood Pressure (mm Hg) *   Diastolic Blood Pressure (mm Hg) ○
[   ]   [   ]
Value must be between 90-200   Value must be between 60-130

Total Cholesterol (mg/dL) *   HDL Cholesterol (mg/dL) *   LDL Cholesterol (mg/dL) ❶ ○
[   ]   [   ]   [   ]
Value must be between 130 - 320 Value must be between 20 - 100   Value must be between 30-300

History of Diabetes? *   Smoker: ❶ *
| Yes | No | | Yes | | Former | | No |

On Hypertension Treatment? *   On a Statin? ❶ ○   On Aspirin Therapy? ❶ ○
| Yes | No | | Yes | No | | Yes | No |

The ASCVD: What's missing?

- **Heavily dependent on age**

- **Too late (Atherosclerosis process starts early!)**

- ASCVD not explained by major risk factors

- No family history (especially family history of premature ASCVD)

- No calcium score data

- No other cholesterol factors other than lipid panel (Lp(a) levels ≥125 nmol/L (≥50 mg/dL) are considered an ASCVD risk-enhancing factor)

Atherosclerosis starts during youth; the earliest lesions can be identified in the arterial beds of most adolescents. Rapid progression of these early lesions occurs in the 3rd and 4th decades of life. This suggests that the optimal age to begin the prevention of atherosclerosis is as young as possible. Earlier studies have suggested that the age at this effect becomes statistically significant is 8 years old. But it is still unknown who would most benefit from more aggressive, pharmacological intervention to lower risk [20].

What are the Current Recommendations from other guidelines?

For low-density lipoprotein (LDL) cholesterol levels in patients with diabetes, the ADA now recommends a target of less than 70 mg/dL or no greater than 55 mg/dL, depending on the individual's cardiovascular risk (note apoB is not factored in) [62]. For people with diabetes aged 40-75 years at increased cardiovascular risk, including those with one or more atherosclerotic risk factors, high-intensity statin therapy is recommended to reduce LDL cholesterol by 50% or more from baseline *and* to a target of less than 70 mg/dL [63]. Also targeting an Lp(a) of < 50 mg/dL is important [64]. Note that risk here should include a number of factors including family history, smoking status, metabolic status, kidney/blood pressure measurements, lipid levels, activity level, race, and diet. In general, the lower the cholesterol and lipids, the better.

Recommended Treatment Goals for LDL, Lp (a) and Apo B levels

	LDL	Lp (a)	Apo B
Very-High Risk	< 50 mg/dl or >50% reduction	< 50 mg/dl	-
High Risk	<70 mg/dl or >50% reduction		< 90 mg/dl
Intermediate risk	<100 mg/dl		<110 mg/dl
Low risk	<116 mg/dl		<130 mg/dl

64-66

Is there a new calculator by the American Heart Association?

There is a new calculator that starts screening at an earlier age which is important, however similar problems persist. It is still dependent on age more than any other factor, does not start early enough, has no family history, and does not include a coronary calcium score and is heavily reliant on cholesterol levels with no involvement of Lp (a) or Apo B. It also removed race, which was an important marker used to assess a patient's individual risk. See appendix for complete calculator [67].

What is a coronary artery calcium (CAC) scoring (CT calcium scoring)?

It is a non-invasive imaging technique used to assess calcium in the arteries that supply blood to the heart (coronary arteries) by CT scanner (no IV, no contrast used). Coronary artery calcium is a marker of atherosclerosis that leads to narrowing of the arteries supplying blood to the heart. CAC can be used to assess risk of developing coronary artery disease which can lead to cardiovascular events including heart attacks. Remember from the cholesterol model that small plaques (20% blockage etc) explode in one second and become 80% (as an example). This is why routine stress testing is unhelpful as it only picks up plaque that is already advanced [68,69].

Who should get a CAC?

Anyone above the age of 40 who does not already have coronary artery disease. It is especially helpful for those at intermediate risk (10-20% on 10 year risk calculators). This should be repeated every 3 years [70]. Please understand that by definition, an elevated calcium score indicates that you have coronary artery disease (CAD) aka plaque in the arteries of your heart. While this book is geared towards prevention of disease (ie. primary prevention), being diagnosed with CAD means that you already have the disease. However, the topics in this book apply to secondary prevention (preventing a disease once it is already present) and are still recommended.

What do the calcium scores mean?

Low Risk (Score: 0-100):
- Score 0: No detectable coronary artery calcification. Generally associated with a very low risk of coronary events in the next 5-10 years, well below 1%.
- Score 1-100: Mild calcification. Suggests a low risk of coronary events, but slightly higher than with a score of 0. The risk of coronary events ranges between 1% to 10% over the next decade, depending on the exact score and patient-specific factors like age and sex.
- Follow what's in this book, usually no need for medications (discuss with your physician).

Medium Risk (Score: 101-400):
- Moderate calcification. Indicates a more significant presence of coronary artery disease. Patients with scores in this range typically have a 10-20% risk of coronary events within the next 10 years.
- Follow what's in this book, plus possible need for medication (discuss with your physician).

High Risk (Score: >400):
- Extensive calcification. Indicates a high likelihood of at least one significant coronary artery obstruction. Patients with scores above 400 are at a high risk of coronary events, with more than a 20% risk of experiencing a coronary event within 10 years.
- Follow what's in this book, high likelihood of needing cholesterol medication (discuss with your physician).

Calcium scoring prognosis:

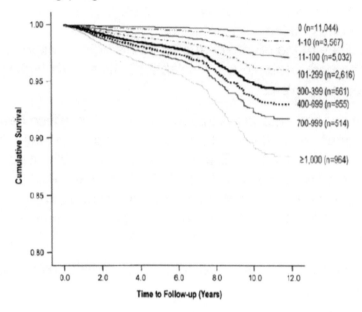

van Werkhoven JM, Bax JJ, Nucifora G, et al. The value of multi-slice-computed tomography coronary angiography for risk stratification. *Journal of Nuclear Cardiology: Official Publication of the American Society of Nuclear Cardiology.* 2009;16(6):970-980. doi:https://doi.org/10.1007/s12350-009-9144-3

Should women get a CAC?

Women were underrepresented in prior risk scores. CAC can help detect early signs of atherosclerosis in women who may not otherwise be identified as high risk. CACs are an excellent screening tool and utilize very low dose radiation compared to other stress testing.

What are the limitations of the CAC?

Previous study showed that the prevalence of noncalcified plaque was 11.1% in patients with no CAC and 23.4% in the mild CAC group (P=0.014). Multiple plaques were detected in 2.6% of the group with no CAC and 3.7% of the group with mild CAC (P=0.59). Significant coronary artery stenosis was found in one patient in the group with no CAC (0.9%) and three patients in the group with mild CAC (2.8%, P=0.35) [71].

Here comes the role of CT coronary angiography:

What is a CT coronary angiogram?

It is a non-invasive imaging technique that uses intravenous contrast to visualize the coronary arteries. It gives detailed images of the arteries which can detect narrowing, blockages and other abnormalities of the coronary arteries. It also differentiates between stable and unstable plaques. Unstable plaques have higher risk for acute coronary events.

CT coronary angiography is the only imaging test which has shown a reduction in CVD mortality and myocardial infarction as demonstrated by SCOT-HEART trial (2.3% vs. 3.9%; hazard ratio, 0.59; 95% confidence interval [CI], 0.41 to 0.84; P=0.004). As it allows more preventive therapies to be initiated earlier (odds ratio, 1.40; 95% CI, 1.19 to 1.65), in addition to more antianginal therapies (odds ratio, 1.27; 95% CI, 1.05 to 1.54) [72].

Ok so how do I actually treat high cholesterol? (Hint: read the rest of the book!)

1. **Diet (see obesity section)**
2. **Exercise (see exercise section)**
3. **Weight loss (see obesity/exercise section)**
4. **Smoking cessation (see smoking section)**
5. **Limit Alcohol (see obesity section)**
6. **Medications**
   - Although there are a lot of treatment options, it is still largely determined by genetics except high triglycerides which can be much more affected by diet. Medications include the statins, Ezetimibe (Zetia), the PSK9 inhibitors, and Bempedoic Acid.

I've heard of Statins! I've also heard bad things about them?

Statins are the most famous class of medications used to lower cholesterol levels, especially LDL. They can also modestly increase HDL levels and reduce triglycerides. Statins have been used in patients with established coronary artery disease, and for those with a high risk of cardiovascular events.

Statin therapy reduced the risk of major coronary events, major cerebrovascular events, and revascularizations by 29.2% (95% CI, 16.7%-39.8%) (P<.001), 14.4% (95% CI, 2.8%-24.6%) (P = .02), and 33.8% (95% CI, 19.6%-45.5%) (P<.001), respectively. Statins produced a nonsignificant reduction in coronary heart disease mortality (22.6%; RR 95% CI, 0.56-1.08; P = 0.13) and overall mortality (RR 0.92; 95% CI, 0.84-1.01) (P = 0.09). There were statistically significant permanent increases in cancer or liver failure [73,74].

The Number Needed to Treat (NNT) to prevent one major vascular event in those at the lowest levels of risk for which statins could be recommended was 40 according to the 1994 and 1998 guidelines (i.e. an ASCVD of 20%); 73 according to the 2004 and 2007 guidelines; and 400 according to the 2012 and 2016 guidelines (i.e. an ASCVD of 7.5%). This means that by today's standards, you would need to treat about 268 people over 5 years to prevent one stroke, and approximately 60 people to prevent one non-fatal heart attack [74,75].

Ok but what about side effects?

Statins are generally well tolerated. Most common side effects are muscle aches (10%) and elevated liver enzymes. It rarely can cause muscle damage called rhabdomyolysis. Statins can cause muscle aches as it inhibits an enzyme in the liver which is also located in the muscles [76]. Coenzyme Q 10 has been used to prevent muscle

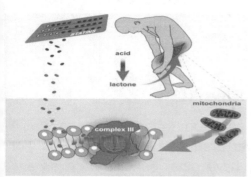

aches associated with statins (although there is no evidence that it works). When you have these side effects it is recommended to just switch to a different statin [77]. Pravastatin works on a different enzyme in the liver and therefore is considered the mildest in terms of side effect profile [78].

Scientists identify mechanism behind statin-induced muscle weakness. www.medicalnewstoday.com. Published September 2, 2015. https://www.medicalnewstoday.com/articles/298911

Do statins cause Diabetes/Insulin Resistance?

The mechanism for statins leading to diabetes is as follows: statins inhibit LDL production, which leads to an increase in LDL receptors on the liver but also the pancreas. This floods the pancreas with

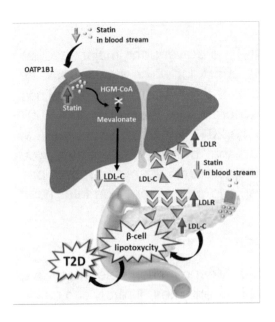

LDL which damages the beta cells that make insulin, leading to decreased insulin and potential risk of diabetes. However, in studies this is only seen at the highest doses of atorvastatin which is 80 mg. The Number Needed to Harm (ie. the number of patients on statins for 5 years to get one case of DM) is about the same as the NNT for a non fatal MI (67). We recommend decreasing statins to the lowest level possible to achieve cholesterol guideline goals. Approximately 85% of that goal is achieved with rosuvastatin 10 mg or atorvastatin 20 mg in most patients [79,80].

Laakso M, Lilian Fernandes Silva. Statins and risk of type 2 diabetes: mechanism and clinical implications. *Frontiers in Endocrinology* 2023;14. doi:https://doi.org/10.3389/fendo.2023.1239335

Do Statins cause Alzheimer's dementia?

Overall Statins have a protective effect on Alzheimer's disease as it decreases triglycerides. However, reducing triglycerides is not enough of an explanation. They have other benefits such as anti inflammatory properties and overall can lead to a reduction in dementia risk [81].

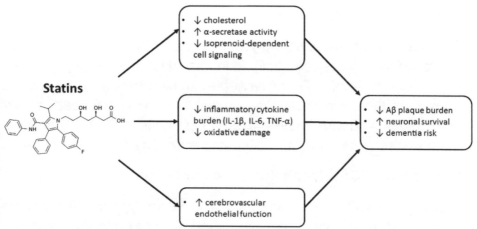

Padala, Kalpana & Potter, Jane & Ikezu, Tsuneya. (2009). HMGCoA-Reductase Inhibitors in Dementia: Benefit or Harm. Clinical Medicine : Geriatrics. 2009.

What about Ezetimibe (Zetia)

Ezetimibe is one of the medications that can lower cholesterol levels by blocking intestinal absorption of the cholesterol in the small intestine. It is usually used as an adjunctive therapy with statins if the target level is not achieved with statins or can be used as monotherapy in patients not tolerating statins [82].
*Overall, there is limited evidence of ezetimibe in primary prevention.

Previous study showed that ezetimibe has improvement in cardiovascular events but this study was done in Japan and included patients > 75 years

- Ezetimibe reduced the incidence of the primary outcome of heart attacks (hazard ratio [HR], 0.66; 95% CI, 0.50–0.86; P=0.002). Regarding the secondary outcomes, the incidences of composite cardiac events (HR, 0.60; 95% CI, 0.37–0.98; P=0.039) and coronary revascularization (HR, 0.38; 95% CI, 0.18–0.79; P=0.007) were lower in the ezetimibe group than in the control group; however, there was no difference in the incidence of stroke, all-cause mortality, or adverse events between trial groups. [83]

What about Fibrates?

Fibrates help break down triglycerides and are mainly used for their reduction, as well as potentially increase HDL, while having a limited effect on LDL/ApoB. There have been mixed results in large scale trials, and therefore these are typically not recommended as first line agents and are mainly used in patients with very elevated triglycerides (think familial hypertriglyceridemia) [84].

What about PCSK9 inhibitors, the injections?

PCSK9 (proprotein convertase subtilisin/kexin type 9) inhibitors are a class of medication that are used to treat high cholesterol, especially when other medications (statins or ezetimibe) were not effective or not tolerated. PCSK9 inhibitors include Evolocumab, and alirocumab. PCSK9 inhibitors are potent inhibitors of LDL receptor degradation which help clear LDL cholesterol from the blood [85, 86].

How does PCSK9 work?

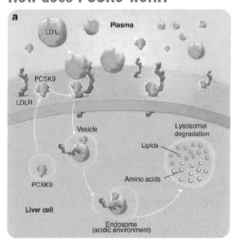

a) Secreted PCSK9 binds to LDLR on the liver cell surface and mediates the lysosomal degradation of the complex formed by PCSK9 - LDLR - LDL.

How does Inhibitors work?

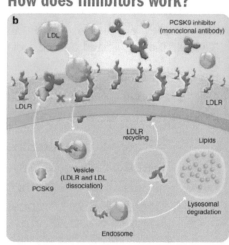

b) In the presence of a monoclonal antibody that binds to PCSK9, the PCSK9-mediated degradation of LDLR is inhibited, resulting in an increased uptake of LDL-cholesterol by LDLR as more LDLR are recycled at the cell surface.

PCSK9 and its Inhibitors: A new approach in lipid lowering therapy | BioVendor R&D. www.biovendor.com. https://www.biovendor.com/pcsk9-and-its-inhibitors-a-new-approach-in-lipid-lowering-therapy

They reduce the level of LDL in addition to a reduction of Lp (a) levels. PCSK9 inhibitors can reduce LDL levels up to 60-70% alone or when used with statins or other cholesterol lowering medications [87].

- Reduction in the level of LDL-C by around 53% [87]

- Reduction of LDL-C by 39% when compared with ezetimibe (Zetia) combined with a statin [87]
- It has also shown a reduction of the risk of cardiovascular events when compared with placebo (OR 0.86, CI 0.8-0.92), and when compared with ezetimibe(Zetia) combined with a statin (OR 0.45, CI 0.3-0.75) [88]

PCSK9 inhibitors are particularly useful in familial hypercholesterolemia (a genetic condition characterized with very high levels of cholesterol that occurs from birth). In the FOURIER trial, Evolocumab showed reduced cardiovascular mortality, myocardial infarction, or urgent revascularization [89]. They are the only known class of medications to significantly reduce Lp(a) by 30-40% (although targeted therapy will be coming out in the next couple of years for this condition) [90,91]. In addition, Evolocumab may also reduce the progression of aortic stenosis and need for aortic valve replacement (?related to Lp(a)) [92]. PCSK9 inhibitors are typically self-administered by subcutaneous injections that are usually given every 2-4 weeks, depending on the specific medication and dosage regimen.

Side effects? None unless specifically allergic to antibody

What about Bempedoic Acid (Nexletol)

- It inhibits an enzyme that is involved in making LDL. It only acts in the liver so diabetes risk is significantly less. The CLEAR study showed that Bempedoic acid showed a mean reduction of LDL 29.2 mg compared with placebo. It showed improvement of composite outcome including MACE, defined as cardiovascular death, nonfatal MI, not fatal stroke or coronary revascularization (11.7% vs 13.3%; HZ, 0.87: 95% CI 0.79-0.96; p=0.004). Bempedoic acid did not show significant effect on stroke, death from cardiovascular causes or all cause death [93].

Side effects: it increases the incidence of gout and gallstones.

Wait, you haven't mentioned HDL once! Doesn't having a high HDL negate any bad cholesterol?

We understand very little about HDL ("good cholesterol") and the complex interactions these particles have in cholesterol transport. While HDL in theory brings cholesterol back to the liver and reduces plaque burden, efforts to raise HDL with CETP inhibitors (an enzyme that when blocked raises HDL) have failed to improve outcomes. Moreover having a high HDL does not negate a high apob/LDL in terms of CVD outcomes. One CETP inhibitor, obicetrapib, one of the strongest ever developed, is showing promise, however there is no outcome data at this time [94].

What about Fish Oil and Omega-3 Fatty acids?

It is an essential nutrient (not produced by our body) and therefore must be obtained from diet. A number of trials have shown that low levels of omega 3 can lead to dementia, anxiety, cognitive decline and cardiovascular events such as heart attacks and strokes. There are several omega-3 fatty acids including ALA (Alpha-Linolenic Acid), EPA (Eicosapentaenoic Acid) and DHA (Docosahexaenoic Acid). Broadly, EPA is used for cardiovascular disease prevention while DHA is used for brain health. ALA is the precursor to EPA and subsequently DHA (but conversion to EPA is more efficient (5-10% conversion vs. DHA which is 2-5%) [95,96].

1. ALA: found mainly in plants including flaxseed, chia seeds, walnut, and echium seed oils
2. EPA: found mainly in fish including salmon, mackerel, sardines, and anchovies.
3. DHA: found mainly in fish including salmon, tuna, sardines, shellfish and herring.

What do omega-3 fatty acids do?

Omega-3 can reduce inflammation, are important for brain function and vision, lower triglyceride levels and can help with reduction of blood pressure.

How do you measure your omega 3 levels?

You can measure it with a blood test or an at home test using a finger prick. The goal is to have levels to as high a dose as possible. The mean omega-3 index of dolphins is 19.9% percent compared with 9% for Japanese people and 5% for Americans [96].

What is the Evidence?

Data is very mixed on the beneficial roles of fish oils in general. The GISSI-Prevenazione Trial in 1999 found that heart attack survivors who took omega 3 lowered their chances of having a fatal heart attack and studies done in 2012 showed that DHA improved brain function in older adults and reduced inflammation. However, only two prior studies (JELIUS and REDUCE-IT) showed the benefit of the EPA only version of fish oil in the reduction of major adverse cardiovascular events and cardiovascular death. Omega-3 administration could be associated with higher risk of gastrointestinal side effects and higher incidence of investigator reported atrial fibrillation (which causes strokes) and bleeding. A Cochrane review in 2018 (amalgamation of all the evidence) showed no benefits of supplemental fish oil on mortality or cardiovascular health (although most trials used much lower doses of fish oil than below). Also, as stated above, fish oil is a PUFA (polyunsaturated fat) which is prone to oxidation (when rancid) which is how the process of plaque formation occurs. A common theme of the only two positive trials of fish oil was that they were EPA only (although DHA is posited to be helpful for brain health) and that the doses were very high (like 4 grams per day!). Overall, we recommend, when possible, to obtain most of your omega 3 from actual fish sources, which has been shown to have benefit in a number of trials without the side effects [94,96-98].

Conclusion

This is the most complicated chapter in the whole book, both for patients and clinicians. In general, screen for hyperlipidemia using a lipid panel (for the triglyceride level), apoB and Lp(a) as early as possible, as these tests are the most accurate way to assess your lipid status. Imaging tests such as calcium scores and coronary CT scans can actually visualize plaque in the arteries of your heart before anything bad happens. Management of hyperlipidemia should include lifestyle modifications including diet, exercise, weight loss, and smoking cessation, in addition to medications. Understand that a lot of this is genetically driven, and more than any other section there is a role for pharmacologic management.

References

1. Cox RA, García-Palmieri MR. Cholesterol, Triglycerides, and Associated Lipoproteins. PubMed. Published 1990. https://www.ncbi.nlm.nih.gov/books/NBK351/#:~:text=Triglycerides%20are%20fatty%20acid%20esters

2. American Heart Association. HDL (good), LDL (bad) cholesterol and triglycerides. American Heart Association. Published November 6, 2020. https://www.heart.org/en/health-topics/cholesterol/hdl-good-ldl-bad-cholesterol-and-triglycerides

3. Why Is Cholesterol Needed by the Body? Healthline. Published December 7, 2018. https://www.healthline.com/health/high-cholesterol/why-is-cholesterol-needed#goals

4. Lichtenstein AH. Triglyceride - an overview | ScienceDirect Topics. www.sciencedirect.com. Published 2013. https://www.sciencedirect.com/topics/agricultural-and-biological-sciences/triglyceride

5. Yi SW, Yi JJ, Ohrr H. Total cholesterol and all-cause mortality by sex and age: a prospective cohort study among 12.8 million adults. Scientific Reports. 2019;9(1). doi:https://doi.org/10.1038/s41598-018-38461-y

6. Yang ST, Kreutzberger AJB, Lee J, Kiessling V, Tamm LK. The role of cholesterol in membrane fusion. Chemistry and Physics of Lipids. 2016;199(1):136-143. doi:https://doi.org/10.1016/j.chemphyslip.2016.05.003

7. Cortes V. Physiological and pathological implications of cholesterol. Frontiers in Bioscience. 2014;19(3):416. doi:https://doi.org/10.2741/4216

8. Cerk IK, Wechselberger L, Oberer M. Adipose Triglyceride Lipase Regulation: An Overview. Current Protein & Peptide Science. 2017;19(2). doi:https://doi.org/10.2174/1389203718666170918160110

9. Mahley RW, Innerarity TL, Rall SC, Weisgraber KH. Plasma lipoproteins: apolipoprotein structure and function. Journal of Lipid Research. 1984;25(12):1277-1294. https://pubmed.ncbi.nlm.nih.gov/6099394/

10. Salter AM, Brindley DN. The biochemistry of lipoproteins. Journal of Inherited Metabolic Disease. 1988;11(S1):4-17. doi:https://doi.org/10.1007/bf01800566

11. Glavinovic T, Thanassoulis G, de Graaf J, Couture P, Hegele RA, Sniderman AD. Physiological Bases for the Superiority of Apolipoprotein B Over Low-Density Lipoprotein Cholesterol and Non–High-Density Lipoprotein Cholesterol as a Marker of Cardiovascular Risk. Journal of the American Heart Association. 2022;11(20). doi:https://doi.org/10.1161/jaha.122.025858

12. Farzam K, Senthilkumaran S. Lipoprotein A. PubMed. Published 2023. https://www.ncbi.nlm.nih.gov/books/NBK570621/#:~:text=The%20desirable%20and%20optimal%20test

13. Mangaraj M, Nanda R, Panda S. Apolipoprotein A-I: A Molecule of Diverse Function. *Indian Journal of Clinical Biochemistry.* 2015;31(3):253-259. doi:https://doi.org/10.1007/s12291-015-0513-1

14. Lipoprotein (a). www.heart.org. https://www.heart.org/en/health-topics/cholesterol/genetic-conditions/lipoprotein-a

15. Huang Y, Mahley RW. Apolipoprotein E: Structure and function in lipid metabolism, neurobiology, and Alzheimer's diseases. *Neurobiology of Disease.* 2014;72:3-12. doi:https://doi.org/10.1016/j.nbd.2014.08.025

16. Qiao YN, Zou YL, Guo SD. Low-density lipoprotein particles in atherosclerosis. *Frontiers in Physiology.* 2022;13. doi:https://doi.org/10.3389/fphys.2022.931931

17. Lipid Metabolism - an overview | ScienceDirect Topics. www.sciencedirect.com. https://www.sciencedirect.com/topics/agricultural-and-biological-sciences/lipid-metabolism#:~:text=Lipid%20metabolism%20involves%20the%20synthesis

18. Loftus I. Mechanisms of Plaque Rupture. PubMed. Published 2011. https://www.ncbi.nlm.nih.gov/books/NBK534259/

19. Bentzon JF, Otsuka F, Virmani R, Falk E. Mechanisms of Plaque Formation and Rupture. *Circulation Research.* 2014;114(12):1852-1866. https://www.ahajournals.org/doi/full/10.1161/CIRCRESAHA.114.302721

20. Gidding SS. Assembling Evidence to Justify Prevention of Atherosclerosis Beginning in Youth. *Circulation.* 2010;122(24):2493-2494.

doi:https://doi.org/10.1161/circulationaha.110.992123

21. Cox RA, García-Palmieri MR. Cholesterol, Triglycerides, and Associated Lipoproteins. Nih.gov. Published 2000. https://www.ncbi.nlm.nih.gov/books/NBK351/

22. Formanowicz D, Radom M, Rybarczyk A, Tanaś K, Formanowicz P. Control of Cholesterol Metabolism Using a Systems Approach. *Biology.* 2022;11(3):430. doi:https://doi.org/10.3390/biology11030430

23. American Heart Association. What Is Cholesterol? www.heart.org. Published November 6, 2020. https://www.heart.org/en/health-topics/cholesterol/about-cholesterol

24. Dehghan M, Mente A, Zhang X, et al. Associations of fats and carbohydrate intake with cardiovascular disease and mortality in 18 countries from five continents (PURE): a prospective cohort study. *The Lancet.* 2017;390(10107):2050-2062. doi:https://doi.org/10.1016/s0140-6736(17)32252-3

25. Telmisartan, Ramipril, or Both in Patients at High Risk for Vascular Events. *New England Journal of Medicine.* 2008;358(15):1547-1559. doi:https://doi.org/10.1056/nejmoa0801317

26. Effects of the angiotensin-receptor blocker telmisartan on cardiovascular events in high-risk patients intolerant to angiotensin-converting enzyme inhibitors: a randomised controlled trial. *The Lancet.* 2008;372(9644):1174-1183. doi:https://doi.org/10.1016/s0140-6736(08)61242-8

27. Sacks FM, Lichtenstein AH, Wu JHY, et al. Dietary Fats and Cardiovascular Disease: A Presidential Advisory From the American Heart Association. *Circulation.* 2017;136(3):e1-e23. doi:https://doi.org/10.1161/CIR.0000000000000510

28. Polyunsaturated Fats. www.heart.org. https://www.heart.org/en/healthy-living/healthy-eating/eat-smart/fats/polyunsaturated-fats#.~:text=Polyunsaturated%20fats%20are%20fat%20molecules

29. Antoni R. Dietary saturated fat and cholesterol: cracking the myths around eggs and cardiovascular disease. *Journal of Nutritional Science.* 2023;12:e97. doi:https://doi.org/10.1017/jns.2023.82

30. The Minnesota Coronary Experiment re-analysis by Ramsden et al is a wake-call to re-evaluate the use of polyunsaturated oils and spreads in modern clinical diets? *wwwbmjcom.* Published online January 20, 2024. https://www.bmj.com/content/353/bmj.i1246/rr-5

31. Hong Y. Framingham Heart Study (FHS) | National Heart, Lung, and Blood Institute (NHLBI). Nih.gov. Published April 16, 2018. https://www.nhlbi.nih.gov/science/framingham-heart-study-fhs

32. Mahmood SS, Levy D, Vasan RS, Wang TJ. The Framingham Heart Study and the epidemiology of cardiovascular disease: a historical perspective. *The Lancet.* 2014;383(9921):999-1008. doi:https://doi.org/10.1016/s0140-6736(13)61752-3

33. Aguib Y, Al Suwaidi J. The Copenhagen City Heart Study (Østerbroundersøgelsen). *Global Cardiology Science & Practice.* 2015;2015(3):33. doi:https://doi.org/10.5339/gcsp.2015.33

34. Friedewald WT, Levy RI, Fredrickson DS. Estimation of the concentration of low-density lipoprotein cholesterol in plasma, without use of the preparative ultracentrifuge. *Clinical Chemistry.* 1972;18(6):499-502. https://pubmed.ncbi.nlm.nih.gov/4337382/

35. Kannan S, Mahadevan S, Ramji B, Jayapaul M, Kumaravel V. LDL-cholesterol: Friedewald calculated versus direct measurement-study from a large Indian laboratory database. *Indian Journal of Endocrinology and Metabolism.* 2014;18(4):502-504. doi:https://doi.org/10.4103/2230-8210.137496

36. Martins J, Steyn N, Rossouw HM, Pillay TS. Best practice for LDL-cholesterol: when and how to calculate. *Journal of Clinical Pathology.* 2023;76(3):145-152. doi:https://doi.org/10.1136/jcp-2022-208480

37. Wolska A, Remaley AT. Measuring LDL-cholesterol. *Current Opinion in Cardiology.* 2020;35(4):1. doi:https://doi.org/10.1097/hco.0000000000000740

38. Duarte Lau F, Giugliano RP. Lipoprotein(a) and its Significance in Cardiovascular Disease: A Review. *JAMA cardiology.* 2022;7(7):760-769. doi:https://doi.org/10.1001/jamacardio.2022.0987

39. Meeusen JW, Donato LJ, Jaffe AS. Should apolipoprotein B replace LDL cholesterol as therapeutic targets are lowered? *Current Opinion in Lipidology.* 2016;27(4):359-366. doi:https://doi.org/10.1097/mol.0000000000000313

40. Barter PJ, Ballantyne CM, Carmena R, et al. Apo B versus cholesterol in estimating cardiovascular risk and in guiding therapy: report of the thirty-person/ten-country panel. 2006;259(3):247-258. doi:https://doi.org/10.1111/j.1365-2796.2006.01616.x

41. Walldius G, Jungner I. Is there a better marker of cardiovascular risk than LDL cholesterol? Apolipoproteins B and A-I – new risk factors and targets for therapy. *Nutrition, Metabolism and Cardiovascular Diseases.* 2007;17(8):565-571. doi:https://doi.org/10.1016/j.numecd.2007.02.010

42. Sniderman AD, Thanassoulis G, Glavinovic T, et al. Apolipoprotein B Particles and Cardiovascular Disease. *JAMA Cardiology.* Published online October 23, 2019. doi:https://doi.org/10.1001/jamacardio.2019.3780

43. Razavi AC, Bazzano LA, He J, et al. Discordantly normal ApoB relative to elevated LDL-C in persons with metabolic disorders: A marker of atherogenic heterogeneity. *American journal of preventive cardiology.* 2021;7:100190-100190. doi:https://doi.org/10.1016/j.ajpc.2021.100190

44. Dorobanțu M, Halațiu VB, Gheorghe-Fronea O, et al. The Association between Apolipoprotein B, Cardiovascular Risk Factors and Subclinical Atherosclerosis—Findings from the SEPHAR National Registry on Hypertension in Romania. *International Journal of Molecular Sciences*. 2023;24(3):2813. doi:https://doi.org/10.3390/ijms24032813

45. Grundy SM, Stone NJ, Bailey AL, et al. 2018 AHA/ACC/AACVPR/AAPA/ABC/ACPM/ADA/AGS/APhA/ASPC/NLA/PCNA Guideline on the Management of Blood Cholesterol. *Circulation*. 2018;139(25). doi:https://doi.org/10.1161/cir.0000000000000625

46. Farzam K, Senthilkumaran S. Lipoprotein A. PubMed. Published 2023. https://www.ncbi.nlm.nih.gov/books/NBK570621/#:~:text=The%20desirable%20and%20optimal%20test

47.Martel J. Lp(a). Quatuor MD. Published July 24, 2023. Accessed May 1, 2024. https://quatuormd.ca/en/lpa/

48. Sahebkar A, Simental-Mendía LE, Pirro M, et al. Impact of ezetimibe on plasma lipoprotein(a) concentrations as monotherapy or in combination with statins: a systematic review and meta-analysis of randomized controlled trials. *Scientific Reports*. 2018;8(1). doi:https://doi.org/10.1038/s41598-018-36204-7

49. A.-D. Koutsogianni, Georgé Liamis, Liberopoulos EN, P.S. Adamidis, Florentin M. Effects of Lipid-Modifying and Other Drugs on Lipoprotein(a) Levels—Potent Clinical Implications. *Pharmaceuticals*. 2023;16(5):750-750. doi:https://doi.org/10.3390/ph16050750

50. Schwartz GG, Steg PG, Szarek M, et al. Alirocumab and Cardiovascular Outcomes after Acute Coronary Syndrome. *New England Journal of Medicine*. 2018;379(22):2097-2107. doi:https://doi.org/10.1056/nejmoa1801174

51. Reeg, Susanne. (2020). What is the role of ApoE variants in ischemic stroke and other age-related complex diseases?. 10.13140/RG.2.2.23487.79529.

52. Liu CC, Kanekiyo T, Xu H, Bu G. Apolipoprotein E and Alzheimer disease: risk, Mechanisms and Therapy. *Nature Reviews Neurology*. 2013;9(2):106-118. doi:https://doi.org/10.1038/nrneurol.2012.263

53. Huang Y, Mahley RW. Apolipoprotein E: Structure and function in lipid metabolism, neurobiology, and Alzheimer's diseases. *Neurobiology of Disease*. 2014;72:3-12. doi:https://doi.org/10.1016/j.nbd.2014.08.025

54. Reiman EM, Arboleda-Velasquez JF, Quiroz YT, et al. Exceptionally low likelihood of Alzheimer's dementia in APOE2 homozygotes from a 5,000-person neuropathological study. *Nature Communications*. 2020;11(1). doi:https://doi.org/10.1038/s41467-019-14279-8

55.Vaezi Z, Amini A. Familial Hypercholesterolemia. PubMed. Published 2020. https://www.ncbi.nlm.nih.gov/books/NBK556009/

56. S S, V B. Familial Hypercholesterolemia--Epidemiology, Diagnosis, and Screening. Current atherosclerosis reports. Published 2015. https://pubmed.ncbi.nlm.nih.gov/25612857/

57.Centers for Disease Control and Prevention. Familial Hypercholesterolemia | CDC. www.cdc.gov. Published March 20, 2020. https://www.cdc.gov/genomics/disease/fh/FH.htm

58. Ghosh S, Kumar A, Pandit K, Chatterjee P, Mukhopadhyay P. Lipid profile in infant. *Indian Journal of Endocrinology and Metabolism*. 2021;25(1):20. doi:https://doi.org/10.4103/ijem.ijem_396_20

59. Jin J. Lipid Disorders: Screening and Treatment. *JAMA*. 2016;316(19):2056-2056. doi:https://doi.org/10.1001/jama.2016.16650

60. Recommendation: Statin Use for the Primary Prevention of Cardiovascular Disease in Adults: Preventive Medication | United States Preventive Services Taskforce. www.uspreventiveservicestaskforce.org. Published August 23, 2022. https://www.uspreventiveservicestaskforce.org/uspstf/recommendation/statin-use-in-adults-preventive-medication

61. American College of Cardiology. ASCVD Risk Estimator. tools.acc.org. Published 2023. https://tools.acc.org/ldl/ascvd_risk_estimator/index.html#

62. ElSayed NA, Grazia Aleppo, Bannuru RR, et al. 10. Cardiovascular Disease and Risk Management: *Standards of Care in Diabetes—2024. Diabetes Care.* 2023;47(Supplement_1):S179-S218. doi:https://doi.org/10.2337/dc24-s010

63. Arnett DK, Blumenthal RS, Albert MA, et al. 2019 ACC/AHA guideline on the primary prevention of cardiovascular disease. *Circulation.* 2019;140(11):e596-e646. doi:https://doi.org/10.1161/cir.0000000000000678

64. Madsen CM, Kamstrup PR, Langsted A, Varbo A, Nordestgaard BG. Lipoprotein(a)-Lowering by 50 mg/dL (105 nmol/L) May Be Needed to Reduce Cardiovascular Disease 20% in Secondary Prevention. *Arteriosclerosis, Thrombosis, and Vascular Biology.* 2020;40(1):255-266. doi:https://doi.org/10.1161/atvbaha.119.312951

65. Apolipoprotein B: Reference Range, Interpretation, Collection and Panels. *eMedicine.* Published online January 24, 2022. Accessed May 2, 2024. https://emedicine.medscape.com/article/2087335-overview?form=fpf

66. Mach F, Baigent C, Catapano AL, et al. 2019 ESC/EAS Guidelines for the Management of dyslipidaemias: Lipid Modification to Reduce Cardiovascular Risk. *European Heart Journal.* 2019;41(1). doi:https://doi.org/10.1093/eurheartj/ehz455

67.

PREVENT™ Online Calculator. professional.heart.org. https://professional.heart.org/en/guidelines-and-statements/prevent-calculator

68. Grundy SM, Stone NJ, Bailey AL, et al. 2018 AHA/ACC/AACVPR/AAPA/ABC/ACPM/ADA/AGS/APhA/ASPC/NLA/PCNA Guideline on the Management of Blood Cholesterol. *Circulation.* 2018;139(25). doi:https://doi.org/10.1161/cir.0000000000000625

69. Nguyen HL, Liu J, Del Castillo M, Shah T. Role of Coronary Calcium Score to Identify Candidates for ASCVD Prevention. *Current Atherosclerosis Reports.* 2019;21(12). doi:https://doi.org/10.1007/s11883-019-0812-8

70. van Werkhoven JM, Bax JJ, Nucifora G, et al. The value of multi-slice-computed tomography coronary angiography for risk stratification. *Journal of Nuclear Cardiology: Official Publication of the American Society of Nuclear Cardiology.* 2009;16(6):970-980. doi:https://doi.org/10.1007/s12350-009-9144-3

71. Iwasaki K, Matsumoto T, Aono H, Furukawa H, Samukawa M. Prevalence of noncalcified coronary plaque on 64-slice computed tomography in asymptomatic patients with zero and low coronary artery calcium. *Canadian Journal of Cardiology.* 2010;26(7):377-380. doi:https://doi.org/10.1016/s0828-282x(10)70419-0

72. SCOT-HEART INVESTIGATORS. Coronary CT Angiography and 5-Year Risk of Myocardial Infarction. *New England Journal of Medicine.* 2018;379(10):924-933. doi:https://doi.org/10.1056/nejmoa1805971

73. Thavendiranathan P. Primary Prevention of Cardiovascular Diseases With Statin Therapy. *Archives of Internal Medicine*. 2006;166(21):2307. doi:https://doi.org/10.1001/archinte.166.21.2307

74. Byrne P, Cullinan J, Gillespie P, Perera R, Smith SM. Statins for primary prevention of cardiovascular disease: modelling guidelines and patient preferences based on an Irish cohort. *British Journal of General Practice*. 2019;69(683):e373-e380. doi:https://doi.org/10.3399/bjgp19X702701

75. Wiggins BS, Saseen JJ, Page RL, et al. Recommendations for Management of Clinically Significant Drug-Drug Interactions With Statins and Select Agents Used in Patients With Cardiovascular Disease: A Scientific Statement From the American Heart Association. *Circulation*. 2016;134(21). doi:https://doi.org/10.1161/cir.0000000000000456

76. Blazing M, Braunwald E, Lemos J de, et al. Effect of statin therapy on muscle symptoms: an individual participant data meta-analysis of large-scale, randomised, double-blind trials. *The Lancet*. 2022;400(10355):832-845. doi:https://doi.org/10.1016/S0140-6736(22)01545-8

77. Chen W, Ochs-Balcom HM, Ma C, Isackson PJ, Vladutiu GD, Luzum JA. Coenzyme Q10 supplementation for the treatment of statin-associated muscle symptoms. *Future Cardiology*. 2022;18(6):461-470. doi:https://doi.org/10.2217/fca-2021-0106

78. Adams SP, Alaeiilkhchi N, Tasnim S, Wright JM. Pravastatin for lowering lipids. *Cochrane Database of Systematic Reviews*. Published online July 9, 2020. doi:https://doi.org/10.1002/14651858.cd013673

79. Karan Nareshbhai Dabhi, Gohil NV, Tanveer N, et al. Assessing the Link Between Statins and Insulin Intolerance: A Systematic Review. *Cureus*. Published online July 17, 2023. doi:https://doi.org/10.7759/cureus.42029

80. Statins in Persons at Low Risk of Cardiovascular Disease. TheNNT. https://thennt.com/nnt/statins-persons-low-risk-cardiovascular-disease/

81. Padala, Kalpana P., et al. "HMGCoA-reductase inhibitors in dementia: benefit or harm." Clinical Medicine Insights: Geriatrics, 12 June 2009, pp. 13+. Gale OneFile: Health and Medicine, link.gale.com/apps/doc/A328852288/HRCA?u=anon~9058d638&sid=googleScholar&xid=26d82471 .

82. Nutescu EA, Shapiro NL. Ezetimibe: A Selective Cholesterol Absorption Inhibitor. *Pharmacotherapy*. 2003;23(11):1463-1474. doi:https://doi.org/10.1592/phco.23.14.1463.31942

83. Ouchi Y, Sasaki J, Arai H, et al. Ezetimibe Lipid-Lowering Trial on Prevention of Atherosclerotic Cardiovascular Disease in 75 or Older (EWTOPIA 75). *Circulation*. 2019;140(12):992-1003. doi:https://doi.org/10.1161/circulationaha.118.039415

84. Staels B, Dallongeville J, Auwerx J, Schoonjans K, Leitersdorf E, Fruchart JC. Mechanism of Action of Fibrates on Lipid and Lipoprotein Metabolism. *Circulation*. 1998;98(19):2088-2093. doi:https://doi.org/10.1161/01.cir.98.19.2088

85. PCSK9 and its Inhibitors: A new approach in lipid lowering therapy | BioVendor R&D. www.biovendor.com. https://www.biovendor.com/pcsk9-and-its-inhibitors-a-new-approach-in-lipid-lowering-therapy

86. Hajar R. PCSK 9 inhibitors: A short history and a new era of lipid-lowering therapy. *Heart Views*. 2019;20(2):74. doi:https://doi.org/10.4103/heartviews.heartviews_59_19

87. Lepor NE, Kereiakes DJ. The PCSK9 Inhibitors: A Novel Therapeutic Target Enters Clinical Practice. *American health & drug benefits*. 2015;8(9):483-489. https://www.ncbi.nlm.nih.gov/pmc/articles/PMC4719137/

88. Choi JY, Na JO. Pharmacological Strategies beyond Statins: Ezetimibe and PCSK9 Inhibitors. *Journal of Lipid and Atherosclerosis*. 2019;8(2):183-191. doi:https://doi.org/10.12997/jla.2019.8.2.183

89. Sabatine MS, Giugliano RP, Keech AC, et al. Evolocumab and Clinical Outcomes in Patients with Cardiovascular Disease. *New England Journal of Medicine*. 2017;376(18):1713-1722. doi:https://doi.org/10.1056/nejmoa1615664

90. Albosta MS, Grant JK, Taub P, Blumenthal RS, Martin SS, Michos ED. Inclisiran: A New Strategy for LDL-C Lowering and Prevention of Atherosclerotic Cardiovascular Disease. *Vascular Health and Risk Management*. 2023;19:421-431. doi:https://doi.org/10.2147/VHRM.S338424

91. Janneke W.C.M. Mulder, Annette M.H. Galema-Boers, Roeters JE. First clinical experiences with inclisiran in a real-world setting. *Journal of Clinical Lipidology*. 2023;17(6):818-827. doi:https://doi.org/10.1016/j.jacl.2023.09.005

92. Bergmark BA, O'Donoghue ML, Murphy SA, et al. An Exploratory Analysis of Proprotein Convertase Subtilisin/Kexin Type 9 Inhibition and Aortic Stenosis in the FOURIER Trial. *JAMA Cardiology*. 2020;5(6):709-709. doi:https://doi.org/10.1001/jamacardio.2020.0728

93. Nissen SE, Lincoff AM, Brennan D, et al. Bempedoic Acid and Cardiovascular Outcomes in Statin-Intolerant Patients. *New England Journal of Medicine*. 2023;388(15). doi:https://doi.org/10.1056/nejmoa2215024

94. John, Hsieh A, Dicklin MR, Ditmarsch M, Davidson MH. Obicetrapib: Reversing the Tide of CETP Inhibitor Disappointments. *Current Atherosclerosis Reports*. 2023;26(2):35-44. doi:https://doi.org/10.1007/s11883-023-01184-1

94. Yokoyama M, Origasa H, Matsuzaki M, et al. Effects of eicosapentaenoic acid on major coronary events in hypercholesterolaemic patients (JELIS): a randomised open-label, blinded endpoint analysis. *The Lancet*. 2007;369(9567):1090-1098. doi:https://doi.org/10.1016/s0140-6736(07)60527-3

95. Bhatt DL, Steg PG, Miller M, et al. Cardiovascular Risk Reduction with Icosapent Ethyl for Hypertriglyceridemia. *New England Journal of Medicine*. 2019;380(1):11-22. doi:https://doi.org/10.1056/nejmoa1812792

96. Gonzalez-Bergner1* CM, Goldstein1 JD, Bossart2 GD, McCarthy3 P, Reif4 JS, McCulloch1 SD. IAAAM 2013. *VINcom*. Published online March 30, 2015. Accessed May 5, 2024. https://www.vin.com/apputil/content/defaultadv1.aspx?pId=11375&id=5768601#:~:text=The%20mean%20omega%2D3%20index

97. Jialal I, Devaraj S, Huet B, Traber M. GISSI-Prevenzione trial. *The Lancet*. 1999;354(9189):1554. doi:https://doi.org/10.1016/s0140-6736(99)90191-5

98. Omega-3 fatty acids for the primary and secondary prevention of cardiovascular disease. www.cochrane.org. Accessed May 5, 2024. https://www.cochrane.org/news/omega-3-fatty-acids-primary-and-secondary-prevention-cardiovascular-disease#:~:text=Of%20the%2086%20included%20trials

Obesity: Metabolic Dysfunction and Diet
By: Eric Lieberman MD, Jonathan Kahan MD

What you need to know:

1. We can estimate metabolic dysfunction in multiple ways. Metabolic dysfunction leads to most cardiovascular diseases.
2. The combination of eating processed foods and lack of exercise is the root cause of metabolic dysfunction
3. A processed food is wrapped in plastic, has a nutrition label, makes a health claim, lasts a long time and has ingredients not found in a standard kitchen. There are relative grades of processing. The less processed the food the better. The dose makes the poison.
4. There are classes of medications that can aid in weight loss which may be an option for you.
5. Exercise breaks down into resistance training (which everyone should do) and cardio. Cardio should be 75% base training (see below) and 25% High Intensity Interval Training (HIIT) training. There is no upper limit to cardio. Aim to train each muscle group at least twice per week with weights/resistance training (see exercise section)
6. Poor sleep may be caused by lack of direct sunlight in the morning, substances such as caffeine and alcohol, and screens, especially phones. Sleep in a cool, dark, and quiet environment. (See sleep, social and miscellaneous section)

Obesity affects more than 40% of Americans today and is a key driver of several disease processes that impact cardiovascular (CVD) risk[1].

Obesity means I have metabolic issues, right? It's like having diabetes, right?

Metabolic abnormalities have a variety of manifestations including obesity, metabolic syndrome, prediabetes and diabetes. There are different definitions for each of these.

A. Obesity = Elevated body mass index (BMI) which is a ratio of your weight over your height squared (kg/m^2):

WHO CLASSIFICATION OF WEIGHT STATUS	
WEIGHT STATUS	BODY MASS INDEX (BMI), kg/m^2
Underweight	<18.5
Normal range	18.5 – 24.9
Overweight	25.0 – 29.9
Obese	≥ 30
Obese class I	30.0 – 34.9
Obese class II	35.0 – 39.9
Obese class III	≥ 40

Stahl, Jonathan M., and Sandeep Malhotra. "[Figure, BMI Chart with Obesity Classifications...]." *Www.ncbi.nlm.nih.gov*, July 2022

Note: This does not distinguish between muscle, fat, bone or body composition in any way[2]

B. Insulin Resistance is a precursor to prediabetes and diabetes. To test accurately would require a glucose clamp, however, we can estimate using the below calculation (Homeostatic Model of Insulin Resistance aka HOMA IR):

HOMA IR = fasting glucose (mg/dL) X fasting insulin (mU/L) / 405

A value >2 = Insulin Resistance[3]

C. Pre Diabetes (preDM) / Diabetes (DM) = Diabetes is further divided into type 1 (where antibodies attack the pancreas and a patient will require insulin) and type 2 diabetes where a patient's lifestyle leads to the disease. Type 1 is outside the scope of this book whereas type 2 is exactly what this book is about (and much more common). There are 3 ways to test to see if a patient has preDM or DM. This is done either with performing an oral glucose tolerance test (OGTT), testing fasting blood glucose, or measuring hemoglobin A1c. OGTT is performed by first testing your blood sugar (aka glucose) level prior to drinking 75 grams of glucose, then testing it one hour and then two hours after. Hemoglobin A1c measures your 3-month average blood glucose.

Test	Normal	Prediabetes	Diabetes
OGTT	<140 mg/dL	≥140 mg/dL to <200 mg/dL	≥200 mg/dL
FPG	<100 mg/dL	≥100 mg/dL to <126 mg/dL	≥126 mg/dL
A1C	<5.7%	≥5.7% to <6.5%	≥6.5%

[4]

Note: HbA1c measures sugar molecules attached to red blood cells. Sugar is sticky, and this is partly how blockages occur in the smallest arteries (ie. microvascular) of the body.

D. Metabolic Syndrome (X) = a cluster of three out of five (3/5) of the following conditions([5]):

Table 8. Clinical Identification of the Metabolic Syndrome

Risk Factor	Defining Level
Abdominal Obesity*	Waist Circumference'
Men	>102 cm (>40 in)
Women	>88 cm (>35 in)
Triglycerides	≥150 mg/dL
HDL cholesterol	
Men	<40 mg/dL
Women	<50 mg/dL
Blood pressure	≥130/>85 mmHg
Fasting glucose	≥110 mg/dL

Note: metabolic syndrome are signs that a patient has impaired metabolism that can lead to diseases of the arteries

What is food?

Food Definition[6]: material containing or consisting of carbohydrates, fats, and proteins used in the body of an animal to sustain growth, repair, and vital processes and to furnish energy (Webster's dictionary)

****Most "food" in the standard American diet (SAD) aka the Western diet does not meet this definition as they do not perform the latter processes****

What is metabolism?

Metabolism[7]: the process of ingesting food, which is made up of protein, fat, carbohydrates, vitamins/minerals and water and breaking them down into amino acids (protein), free fatty acids (fat), glucose (carbohydrates). This is the catabolism part of metabolism. The next process is anabolism, which is using the basic building blocks of amino acids etc to make up components of the cell eg. enzymes (proteins), membranes (fats) and ATP (glucose/fats). [this is a simplified definition]

Can I be obese but metabolically healthy?

Yes! About 30% of obese patients (as defined by BMI, see above) are considered metabolically healthy[8]. While definitions vary, generally these are patients with normal HOMA-IR (<2, see above) and do not meet Metabolic Syndrome X criteria. HOWEVER, obesity is the root cause of a multitude of other diseases including obstructive sleep apnea (which causes hypertension and fatigue secondary to a buildup of carbon dioxide which is a poison), hypertension, joint and back pain, elevated cholesterol, and coronary artery disease and strokes (this is not an exhaustive list of issues). The higher the weight, the higher the chance of becoming metabolically unhealthy. This is related to the 3 different types of fat and the consequences of fat distribution (see below):

Are there different types of body fat?

Yes! There are 3 main types of fat on a person's body (this is a simplification)[9]:

1. Subcutaneous fat[10], fat that is present around the hips, butt and thighs. Humans can store about ~20 lbs of fat in these areas. These fat cells accept free fatty acids (FFA) and store them within cells in vacuoles (think giant bubbles). When these bubbles burst, they spill FFA into the bloodstream and surrounding tissues which can lead to metabolic syndrome (see below). The way this happens is by FFA entering muscle cells causing sugar regulation dysfunction (muscle is the main regulator of sugar in the body!).
2. Visceral (VAT) fat[11]: This is fat that surrounds organs or has direct access to organs. The most concerning examples of this are abdominal fat and epicardial (beside the heart) fat. Whether the body makes visceral vs. subcutaneous fat appears to be poorly understood, and is a combination of age, genetics, hormonal (estrogen and testosterone) and the lifestyle factors listed in this book. Alcohol may have a predilection for the development of visceral fat. Visceral fat is hormonally active and is a major driver of inflammation. The mechanism where visceral fat leads to metabolic syndrome is via cytokines (signaling chemicals) that increase inflammation in the body, vessels walls and organs, leading to metabolic dysfunction and atherosclerosis (plaque in the arteries of the heart). FFA/cytokines from visceral fat in the abdomen goes straight to the liver via the portal vein (think super highway), causing nonalcoholic fatty liver disease (NAFLD). Epicardial fat sits directly on top of the heart[12]. We can see and measure epicardial fat on ultrasounds of the heart. This type of fat damages the heart in the same way abdominal fat damages the liver. There is a strong correlation between epicardial fat and heart attacks.
3. Organ fat[13], i.e. fat that develops within the organs themselves. Examples of this include fat deposition within

the liver and muscle. You need very little of this fat (less than 1 lbs) to cause issues. Excess sugar, especially fructose, gets converted in the liver to FFA and stored as triglycerides (TG), leading to the development of fatty liver disease and inflammation.

How does obesity lead to metabolic syndrome?

When we consume excess foods that lead to metabolic derangement eg. processed foods, we accumulate excess energy in the form of free fatty acids (FFA)/sugars into the types of fat listed above[14]. If the FFA is stored in subcutaneous fat, then it can spill over leading to inflammation, toxicity, mitochondrial dysfunction and insulin resistance. If the FFA are stored in visceral fat (remember a number of factors play into why excess energy goes into subcutaneous vs. visceral fat including age, genetics etc.) then it can directly damage the organs it is attached to (epicardial fat in the case of the heart, abdominal fat via the portal vein superhighway in the case of the liver). Once these organs uptake the fat e.g. heart, muscle, liver, the FFA cause direct damage to a number of processes leading to overt disease. In the liver they can be stored as triglycerides which cause all the problems discussed above, in the muscle they impair glucose transport (our muscles are the main sinks for sugar) leading to metabolic dysfunction and some are incorporated into the lipoproteins which cause damage to the vascular walls themselves (leading to inflammation and plaque development). Excess sugars can go to the liver where they are converted to triglycerides which then follows the exact mechanisms as above, or leads to chronically elevated insulin which can lead to insulin resistance on its own.

Cause of Obesity AKA Metabolic Syndrome AKA preDM AKA DM

Obesity etc. is a modern problem, rising to epidemic proportions in the 1970's and spreading throughout the rest of the world. The rise of metabolic syndrome and cardiovascular disease correlates with the move to processed and ultra processed foods in combination with lack of activity[15,16]. This leads to most cardiovascular diseases which as previously shown is the number one cause of morbidity and mortality in the world.

What is processed food and why is it bad?

Humans have been processing food for millennia. You can change food without changing macros, but by changing characteristics you can take a food from natural to ultra processed (think apple to applesauce to fruit strip)[17]. Note, I have not changed the macro components at all. The protein, fat and carbohydrates are exactly the same. However, this new form of food has significant consequences. The more processing done to a food, the faster it speeds through our digestive system, which causes us to eat more. Additionally, they are more calorie dense and contain obesogens (chemicals that cause obesity). Furthermore, fiber and other nutrients have an architecture, which are destroyed in the process (more on that later)[18]. It is very important to understand that this is unrelated to macros. It is not about high protein, low carb, fat free, high fiber etc. it is about how close to how the food would exist in nature.

Example: In Keto 1.0 (where no keto friendly i.e. zero carb processed foods were available), people lost a lot of weight and corrected the metabolic issues plaguing them. The main problem with Keto 1.0 was that it was not sustainable in the long term. Now there is keto 2.0 which contains keto pizza, ice cream etc. and people who eat these foods have the same problems as people who eat processed foods despite eating zero carbs.

How can I tell what is processed food?

Approximately 80% of food in our grocery stores in the Western world is processed and our nutritional labels do little to tell us which foods are processed or what was done to them. In general, if it comes in a plastic wrapper or bag it is processed. If it contains ingredients not found in a typical kitchen it is ultra processed. If it makes a health claim such as "high in fiber/vitamins" there is a reasonable chance it is processed. If it has multiple ingredients it is processed. If it has ANY added sugars or sweeteners it is processed (note, there are multiple words for sugar, and on food labels they separate them out, but when added together they make up a large percentage of that food). If a food lasts for a long time (e.g. bread with expiration dates of months, cold cuts etc.) it is highly processed. This is also true if a food is ready to eat (e.g. instant noodles, hot dogs, microwaveable meals). There is a classification system called NOVA[19] which helps break food into 4 categories of processed foods, although at the time of this writing it does not contain every brand/food available. There is a free app called Yuka® which you can scan almost every product to see if it has hazardous chemicals, although at the time of this writing it does not classify foods based on NOVA or state their processing. Note the nutrition label contains very little about what was actually done to our food (and serves as a warning that the food is probably processed). A large proportion of restaurant/fast food is highly processed regardless of health claims.

What about Time Restricted Eating AKA Intermittent Fasting?

Time restricted eating (TRE) (AKA Intermittent Fasting (IF) for the purpose of this book) is one option to maintain a healthy weight and has numerous beneficial cardiovascular effects including decrease in weight, body fat percentage, hypertension, lipid management and blood glucose[20]. TRE works by creating a calorie deficit essentially, in that a person is unable to eat more calories in a smaller window of time. In TRE/IF, a feeding window of 8, 10 or 12 hours is created where all calories are consumed regardless of source. The most studied is an 8-hour eating window with a 16-hour fasting window. Water, black coffee and/or tea (without any additions) appear to not break a fast. The clock starts when first consumption of calories is taken in. Note in the sleep section we are recommending stopping the last consumption of calories 2 hours prior to sleep. We recommend TRE/IF in most patients. Note no significant differences have been observed in hypoglycemia/adverse events in diabetic patients, and the opposite is true, that lower A1c and improved glucose management has been observed. Lastly, if you have trouble obtaining your protein goals (see below), you can have a scoop of protein powder as the benefit outweighs the caloric/fast breaking risk.

Is a calorie a calorie?

In terms of common understanding, the question is if I eat 100 calories worth of food will I absorb 100 calories of that food[21]? The answer is yes if it's processed and no if it is not processed. If you eat 100 calories of almonds you will absorb 70 calories, the rest goes to your gut microbiome (more on that later). Essentially, by doing our digestions for us, a processed food ensures all of our calories are absorbed with maximum efficiency.

But what about low carb, high fat, low fat etc diets?

In Keto 1.0, patients were able to lose weight because there were no processed foods that contained zero carbohydrates. Now in Keto 2.0 there are keto cookies, ice cream, pizza etc. and people are gaining weight back the same as before. The Tsimane tribe in South America are an uncontacted tribe that have no known heart disease and arc considered to have the healthiest hearts in the world[22]. They eat a diet that is 65-70% carbohydrates composed of white rice, yuka, chocolate etc. They violate every major macro diet e.g. low carb and yet have no heart disease. It is not about the macros. Autopsy data from Alaskan Inuit in the 1950's showed less than one fifth the cardiovascular disease of the general population at the time (which was already much lower than it is today)[23]. Their diet consisted mainly of protein and fat. The macros do not matter (much).

But what about protein?

Protein is broken down into amino acids which are the building blocks for structures such as enzymes in our bodies. As such they typically do not contribute to our overall energy balance. HOWEVER, the recommended daily allowance (RDA) for protein is only 0.8 grams/kilogram (a kilogram is 2.2 pounds)[24]. This is to prevent starvation and is entirely too low for optimal health. As such we recommend (unless you have significant kidney disease) approximately **1.5 grams per kilogram of body weight of protein intake per day (0.7 grams per pound of body weight).** Note: this is protein from actual food. Also note you can build muscle just by eating protein, and that the ability of muscle to incorporate protein declines over time (likely from inactivity and not from intrinsic aging)[25].

What about cookies, pizza, ice cream etc?

One can enjoy an occasional "treat" such as a cookie, pizza or ice cream. Consuming a diet that contains a large percentage of "unprocessed" foods but allowing small amounts of "processed" foods is acceptable and can be part of a healthy lifestyle. It is a matter of balance. Bear in mind that it does take planning and effort to achieve this balance, particularly understanding the high prevalence of processed food that we encounter routinely in the grocery aisle and at most restaurants."

What about fast food/restaurants?

The vast majority of fast food and restaurant food is processed food. For example, in Europe, the bread in fast food restaurants is actually listed as cake (!) and multiple chains were caught using mattress chemicals in their breads (azodicarbonamide)[26]. Most foods in fast food and restaurants are highly processed. In a number of states, the restaurants can be worse, as the fast food industry has to publish their nutritional information (although nothing about how they process the food which is the whole point). The impact of public-school nutrition on our children is significant, potentially contributing to the epidemic of childhood obesity. More importantly we are missing the opportunity to provide a solid foundation to our children for good nutritional habits for them to build upon as they mature. We recommend avoiding fast food/restaurants where possible, however we understand that socializing occurs frequently in these locations; which is a good thing (see social/misc section)! Therefore, to limit the damage, we recommend consuming a small high protein/fat meal e.g. a bowl of greek yogurt prior to the meal. That way you can order whatever you would like and just eat less of it.

What about saturated fat intake?

Saturated fat is found in animal and dairy products and some plant products such as coconuts and palm oils. Once ingested they can go to the liver and raise the LDL cholesterol (see cholesterol chapter). Some studies suggest insulin resistance as well[27]. The mechanism of insulin resistance may be related to lipid intermediates that accumulate in muscle cells (the main regulator and storage of sugars) leading to insulin resistance. However, two very well-done studies in the 1970's (the Minnesota Coronary Experiment[28] and the Sydney Diet Heart Study[29]) showed that replacing saturated fat with polyunsaturated fat (i.e. vegetable oil/linoleic acid) led to higher mortality. For every 1% increase in energy from polyunsaturated fats there was a 17% increase in death. Overall, at this time we feel context matters, and the recommendation is to not limit or follow saturated vs. unsaturated fats, but instead to focus on high quality, unprocessed foods as above, still in the right way to proceed.

*** Caveat: Approximately 1 out of 250 of you reading this have Familial Hyperlipidemia (FH) [see cholesterol section][30]. The treatment for this is a low saturated fat diet! The mechanism is likely related to over stimulation of lipids, specifically LDL in FH, which is exacerbated by saturated fat. Get your ApoB tested!

What about Alcohol?

One Beer (12 0z) = 1 glass of wine (5 oz) = 1 shot of distilled alcohol (1.5 oz). One standard drink is 14 grams of Ethanol. There is no safe level of alcohol consumption for the heart[31]. It leads to cardiovascular disease, hypertension, strokes, arrhythmias and addiction. It is calorie dense and leads to weight gain secondary to alteration in the hormones that regulate hunger and satiety (ghrelin and leptin). Alcohol causes inflammation, reactive oxygen species (aka free radicals), neurocognitive deficits and leaky gut/inflammation. There have been studies showing the benefits of moderate consumption of alcohol, particularly red wine. This recommendation is found in the Mediterranean diet and in the French paradox, where it is observed that French citizens live longer than Americans despite high levels of smoking and saturated fat (although see above)[32]. It is thought to be secondary to red wine consumption which contains resveratrol, however you would need to drink around 400 liters of red wine a day to get 1 gram of resveratrol (note we do not endorse resveratrol either). When broken down by region, the higher red wine consumers in France also ate more fruits and vegetables, negating the effects of red wine itself. An alternative explanation to the French Paradox is less processed food eating overall (healthier) and a more social component to alcohol use. Again, like processed foods, sugar etc. the dose makes the poison. Overall, we follow the Canadian guidelines of 2 standard drinks maximum per week[33]. What's the point you ask? Indeed.

What about water?

Recommendations for the amount of water that should be consumed on a daily basis vary, however, a general rule is to aim for drinking enough water to have clear or slightly yellow urine and aim for one liter of water extra per hour of exercise. Do not consume water from plastic bottles (see microplastic section).

What about artificial sweeteners?

Artificial sweeteners lead to weight gain by activating the pancreas and digestive system via sweet receptors in the tongue[34]. When no calories are detected, these organ systems send signals to the brain to seek out calories rather than shut down. Additionally, they affect the gut microbiome (see below) in ways that we do not understand[35]. Some appear safe such as Xylitol which may block strep mutans proliferation in the oral cavity (the bacteria that causes cavities) while others such as Aspartame are now being labeled as a potential carcinogen[36,37]. The research is evolving in this area and at this time we cannot recommend use of artificial sweeteners.

What about fiber?

Fiber has a complex architecture, which is why you cannot process fiber and put it into food. There are two types of fiber, soluble and insoluble. Soluble fiber forms a gel and coats the digestive tract. It comes from whole wheat (not processed), fruits such as apples and vegetables such as carrots (you can search up a more exhaustive list). Insoluble fiber forms a scaffold and adds bulk to stool, preventing constipation and comes from beans, nuts and seeds. These two sources of fiber interact with our gut microbiome (see below) to lead to weight loss, reduced calorie absorption (through coating the intestines) and improved insulin sensitivity. Fiber is a main prebiotic (see below) which allows bacteria to ferment and produce short chain fatty acids (SCFAs) which have many beneficial effects such as reduced inflammation (inflammation is a precursor to cardiovascular disease), metabolism satiety (interaction with L cells of intestine to create GLP-1, see below), and maintaining gut barrier integrity[38]. Some individuals experience gastrointestinal discomfort or bloating from excess fiber ingestion, which can be severe. We recommend gradually increasing your fiber intake (of both kinds and from natural sources) until you begin to feel GI discomfort and then lower the dose to the maximally tolerated (aim for 25-35 grams per day, but you must be able to tolerate it!)[39].

What about probiotics?

Probiotics are living beneficial (aka good) microbes, prebiotics are food for these microbes eg. fermented foods [Kimchi, pickled foods] and fiber (see above), and post biotics are the beneficial compounds procedure by these probiotics. Most probiotics purchased in supplement form (on shelves, not refrigerated, not in food) are DOA (dead on arrival)[40]. There are a few companies that are at least proven to be alive on arrival (look for ones that come refrigerated and have actual studies). Moreover, since probiotics are considered, a supplement there is no regulation on the type, quantity, dosing, or health outcomes associated with ingestion of these. Unprocessed Greek yogurt which contains these probiotics appears to be beneficial in appetite regulation, and even can lead to the reduction in the risk of type II diabetes[41]. In theory, certain species such as Akkermansia will interact with L cells of the intestines to tell the pancreas to release GLP-1, while simultaneously altering the absorption of various nutrients (see below)[42]. Furthermore, we know transplanting the microbiome from an obese to a thin mouse can cause the thin mouse to become obese[43]. The gut microbiome can also affect inflammation through lipopolysaccharide production (which is bad) and reactive oxygen species scavenging (a common pathway with atheroma aka plaque formation in the arteries). We believe this (and above, see fiber section) are the reason why fiber has been proven to have beneficial cardiovascular outcomes. More research is needed in this area before recommendations on specific probiotics can be made, although the literature looks promising and will be an area of future advancement in the field of preventive cardiology.

What about Atrial Fibrillation?

Atrial fibrillation is the most common arrhythmia in the world and approximately 25% of all strokes come from atrial fibrillation!!!! As of 12/2023 the atrial fibrillation guidelines have listed weight loss as a class 1 (highest level) of recommendation for any patient with a BMI > 27 kg/m2) with an ideal target of 10% weight loss[44].

What about pharmacotherapy for obesity?

Over the past few years there has been an explosion in the use of pharmacotherapy for obesity. The two most commonly prescribed medications currently are Ozempic (for diabetics) = Wegovy (for non-diabetics) = Semaglutide [they are the same molecule][45] and Mounjaro (for diabetics) = Zepbound (for non-diabetics) = Tirzepetide [they are the same molecule][46]. Semaglutide is a full agonist (meaning full activator) of glucagon-like peptide -1 (GLP-1) in the pancreas whereas Tirzepetide is a partial agonist of both GLP-1 and GIP. There are going to be several variations of these medications coming on the market but for now we will focus on these two. The basic mechanism of these medications is to slow the digestion of food motility aka slow the speed of food going through the digestive tract and interact in the brain to decrease hunger in ways that are poorly understood[47]. Note that they do not bind sugars. Note also that if GLP-1 agonists slow gut motility and lead to weight loss then the opposite must be true, that foods that speed through the digestive tract i.e. processed foods must lead to weight gain.

These medications have extensive benefits in terms of cardiovascular outcomes, including decreases in weight, insulin resistance, HbA1c, blood sugar, hypertension, cholesterol levels and secondary cardiac outcomes such as prevention of heart attacks and strokes. Secondly, the 4th leading cause of death in America is medication interactions, and because of the improvements in the above, it allows patients to come off of other medications. Thirty six percent of patients in the USA take > 5 medications, and the odds of a drug-drug interaction are 100% at 8 medications[48].

However, there are several significant downsides to these medications including cost ($1400/month in some cases!), supply issues, gastrointestinal side effects (at 10-16% range, nausea and constipation most common), gastroparesis (paralysis of the stomach motility which is reversible), bacterial overgrowth syndrome, weight gain upon discontinuation (see below for mitigation protocol), medication interactions (poorly understood), decreased fluid intake (maybe beneficial in case of alcohol abuse), pancreatitis, medullary thyroid carcinoma, and dissociation (most serotonin is stored in gut, maybe related to the effectiveness of the medication?). Tolerance may develop leading to higher dosing requirements. Furthermore, they may also lead to worsening sarcopenia (muscle loss, which we consider the most serious common side effect) where these medications cause equal loss of fat, bone, muscle and connective tissue.

Often, patients are either too debilitated or too addicted to processed foods/alcohol to begin to exercise and diet seriously. Furthermore, studies back fast initial weight loss in terms of greater weight reduction and long-term maintenance, and patients who utilize fast weight loss protocols are not more susceptible to weight regain than more gradual weight loss[49]. In other words, casinos are popular for a reason!

We begin by determining if a patient is appropriate for pharmacotherapy (you must check with your doctor). It is important to offer a non-pharmacotherapy option as well, so a patient can decide. We typically utilize BMI >27 kg/m2 and one cardiac risk factor such as hypertension or diabetes (in addition to other patient characteristics on an individualized basis). There are also multiple drug interactions and caveats that you and your physician must discuss before initiating.

Our protocol is individualized and is based on the following: early introduction of weightlifting/resistance training, frequent follow ups for titration and side effect assessment, teaching the tools in this book to change lifestyle and behavior (including processed food elimination, TRE, sleep and foundational exercise introduction), followed by a gradual off titration. We utilize DEXA scanning and regular bloodwork to follow muscle mass, visceral fat quantification and multiple other parameters at specified intervals to avoid sarcopenia and other risks/medication interactions. We have seen success in this manner with patients maintaining profound weight losses over more than 18 months.

It is important to note that at this time, the long-term outcomes/side effects of these medications are unknown. It will take many years to understand the full effects of these medications, while newer and different peptide agents will be coming out in the market which may have different properties. You must work with a health care provider who is knowledgeable about the risks and benefits of this class of medications, is willing and able to follow you closely, and have an individualized approach to care. We believe that this will ensure a safe approach to maximize the benefits of this class of medications while minimizing the long-term risks, and at the same time introducing the core principles of preventive cardiology to the patient.

References

1. Alhomoud, Ibrahim S, et al. "Effect of Pharmacist Interventions on the Management of Overweight and Obesity: A Systematic Review." *Journal of the American Pharmacists Association*, 1 Feb. 2024, pp. 102058–102058, https://doi.org/10.1016/j.japh.2024.102058.
2. Stahl, Jonathan M., and Sandeep Malhotra. "[Figure, BMI Chart with Obesity Classifications...]." *Www.ncbi.nlm.nih.gov*, 25 July 2022, www.ncbi.nlm.nih.gov/books/NBK513285/figure/article-35323.image.f1/
3. Salgado, Ana Lúcia Farias de Azevedo, et al. "Insulin Resistance Index (HOMA-IR) in the Differentiation of Patients with Non-Alcoholic Fatty Liver Disease and Healthy Individuals." *Arquivos de Gastroenterologia*, vol. 47, no. 2, 2010, pp. 165–9, www.ncbi.nlm.nih.gov/pubmed/20721461, https://doi.org/10.1590/s0004-28032010000200009.
4. Florida, Kiran Panesar, BPharmS (Hons), MRPharmS, RPh, CPh Consultant Pharmacist and Freelance Medical Writer Orlando. "Prediabetes Management." *Www.uspharmacist.com*, www.uspharmacist.com/article/prediabetes-management-44469.

5. "Health 101 Metabolic Syndrome." *Www.scymed.com*, www.scymed.com/en/smnxdg/health101/edzr/edzr9610_tb8.htm.

6. "Food, N. Meanings, Etymology and More | Oxford English Dictionary." *Oed.com*, 2023, www.oed.com/dictionary/food_n?tab=meaning_and_use, https://doi.org/10.1093//OED//7910243951.

7. Sánchez López de Nava, Arturo, and Avais Raja. "Physiology, Metabolism." *PubMed*, StatPearls Publishing, 12 Sept. 2022, www.ncbi.nlm.nih.gov/books/NBK546690/.

8. Damiri, Basma, et al. "Metabolic Syndrome among Overweight and Obese Adults in Palestinian Refugee Camps." *Diabetology & Metabolic Syndrome*, vol. 10, no. 1, 19 Apr. 2018, https://doi.org/10.1186/s13098-018-0337-2.

9. Thomas, E.L., et al. "Whole Body Fat: Content and Distribution." *Progress in Nuclear Magnetic Resonance Spectroscopy*, vol. 73, Aug. 2013, pp. 56–80, https://doi.org/10.1016/j.pnmrs.2013.04.001.

10. Pinkhasov, Boris B., et al. "Metabolic Syndrome in Men and Women with Upper or Lower Types of Body Fat Distribution." *Health*, vol. 04, no. 12, 2012, pp. 1381–1389, https://doi.org/10.4236/health.2012.412a200.

11. Bergman, Richard N., et al. "Why Visceral Fat Is Bad: Mechanisms of the Metabolic Syndrome." *Obesity*, vol. 14, no. 2S, Feb. 2006, pp. 16S19S, https://doi.org/10.1038/oby.2006.277.

12. Iacobellis, Gianluca. "Epicardial Adipose Tissue in Contemporary Cardiology." *Nature Reviews Cardiology*, 16 Mar. 2022, https://doi.org/10.1038/s41569-022-00679-9. Accessed 22 May 2022.

13. Lim, Jung Sub, et al. "The Role of Fructose in the Pathogenesis of NAFLD and the Metabolic Syndrome." *Nature Reviews Gastroenterology & Hepatology*, vol. 7, no. 5, 6 Apr. 2010, pp. 251–264, https://doi.org/10.1038/nrgastro.2010.41.

14. Suiter, Chase, et al. "Free Fatty Acids: Circulating Contributors of Metabolic Syndrome." *Cardiovascular & Hematological Agents in Medicinal Chemistry*, vol. 16, no. 1, 2018, pp. 20–34, pubmed.ncbi.nlm.nih.gov/29804539/, https://doi.org/10.2174/1871525716666180528100002. Accessed 18 Aug. 2023.

15. Lustig, Robert H. "Ultraprocessed Food: Addictive, Toxic, and Ready for Regulation." *Nutrients*, vol. 12, no. 11, 5 Nov. 2020, p. 3401, www.ncbi.nlm.nih.gov/pmc/articles/PMC7694501/, https://doi.org/10.3390/nu12113401.

16. Golbidi, Saeid, et al. "Exercise in the Metabolic Syndrome." *Oxidative Medicine and Cellular Longevity*, 5 July 2012, www.hindawi.com/journals/omcl/2012/349710/.

17. Lustig, Robert et al (2021). Metabolical: the lure and the lies of processed food, nutrition, and modern medicine. Harper publishing.

18. Chen, J. P., Chen, G. C., Wang, X. P., Qin, L., & Bai, Y. (2017). Dietary fiber and metabolic syndrome: a meta-analysis and review of related mechanisms. *Nutrients*, 10(1), 24.

19. Petrus, R. R., do Amaral Sobral, P. J., Tadini, C. C., & Gonçalves, C. B. (2021). The NOVA classification system: a critical perspective in food science. *Trends in Food Science & Technology*, 116, 603-608.

20. Furmli, S., Elmasry, R., Ramos, M., & Fung, J. (2018). Therapeutic use of intermittent fasting for people with type 2 diabetes as an alternative to insulin. *Case Reports, 2018*, bcr-2017.

21. Nishi, S. K., Kendall, C. W., Bazinet, R. P., Hanley, A. J., Comelli, E. M., Jenkins, D. J., & Sievenpiper, J. L. (2021, September). Almond bioaccessibility in a randomized crossover trial: Is a calorie a calorie?. In *Mayo Clinic Proceedings* (Vol. 96, No. 9, pp. 2386-2397). Elsevier.

22. Thompson, R. C., Thomas, G. S., Neuneubel, A. D., Mahadev, A., Trumble, B., Seabright, E., ... & Kaplan, H. (2023). Atherosclerosis in Indigenous Tsimane: A Contemporary Perspective.

23. DiNicolantonio, James J, and James O'Keefe. "Markedly Increased Intake of Refined Carbohydrates and Sugar Is Associated with the Rise of Coronary Heart Disease and Diabetes among the Alaskan Inuit." *Open Heart*, vol. 4, no. 2, Nov. 2017, p. e000673, https://doi.org/10.1136/openhrt-2017-000673. Accessed 15 Nov. 2019.

24. Phillips, S. M., Chevalier, S., & Leidy, H. J. (2016). Protein "requirements" beyond the RDA: implications for optimizing health. *Applied Physiology, Nutrition, and Metabolism, 41*(5), 565-572.

25. Weijzen, M. E., Kouw, I. W., Geerlings, P., Verdijk, L. B., & van Loon, L. J. (2020). During hospitalization, older patients at risk for malnutrition consume< 0.65 grams of protein per kilogram body weight per day. *Nutrition in Clinical Practice, 35*(4), 655-663.

26. Che, W., Sun, L., Zhang, Q., Zhang, D., Ye, D., Tan, W., ... & Dai, C. (2017). Application of visible/near-infrared spectroscopy in the prediction of azodicarbonamide in wheat flour. *Journal of food science, 82*(10), 2516-2525.

27. Funaki, M. (2009). Saturated fatty acids and insulin resistance. *The journal of medical investigation, 56*(3, 4), 88-92.

28. Ramsden, C. E., Zamora, D., Majchrzak-Hong, S., Faurot, K. R., Broste, S. K., Frantz, R. P., ... & Hibbeln, J. R. (2016). Re-evaluation of the traditional diet-heart hypothesis: analysis of recovered data from Minnesota Coronary Experiment (1968-73). *bmj, 353*.

29. Ramsden, C. E., Zamora, D., Leelarthaepin, B., Majchrzak-Hong, S. F., Faurot, K. R., Suchindran, C. M., ... & Hibbeln, J. R. (2013). Use of dietary linoleic acid for secondary prevention of coronary heart disease and death: evaluation of recovered data from the Sydney Diet Heart Study and updated meta-analysis. *Bmj, 346*, e8707.

30. Padda, I. S., Fabian, D., & Johal, G. S. (2023). Familial Combined Hyperlipidemia.

31. Díaz, L. A., Fuentes-López, E., Idalsoaga, F., Ayares, G., Corsi, O., Arnold, J., ... & Arab, J. P. (2024). Association between public health policies on alcohol and worldwide cancer, liver disease and cardiovascular disease outcomes. *Journal of Hepatology, 80*(3), 409-418.

32. Hu, F. B. (2005). Overweight and increased cardiovascular mortality: no French paradox. *Hypertension, 46*(4), 645-646.

33. "Canada's Guidance on Alcohol and Health | Canadian Centre on Substance Use and Addiction." *Www.ccsa.ca*, www.ccsa.ca/canadas-guidance-alcohol-and-health#:~:text=2%20standard%20drinks%20or%20less. Accessed 8 May 2024.

34. Brown, R. J., De Banate, M. A., & Rother, K. I. (2010). Artificial sweeteners: a systematic review of metabolic effects in youth. *International Journal of Pediatric Obesity, 5*(4), 305-312.

35. Suez, J., Korem, T., Zilberman-Schapira, G., Segal, E., & Elinav, E. (2015). Non-caloric artificial sweeteners and the microbiome: findings and challenges. *Gut microbes, 6*(2), 149-155.

36. Söderling, E. M., Ekman, T. C., & Taipale, T. J. (2008). Growth inhibition of Streptococcus mutans with low xylitol concentrations. *Current microbiology, 56*, 382-385.

37. Landrigan, P. J., & Straif, K. (2021). Aspartame and cancer—new evidence for causation. *Environmental Health, 20*, 1-5.

38. Viuda-Martos, M., López-Marcos, M. C., Fernández-López, J., Sendra, E., López-Vargas, J. H., & Pérez-Álvarez, J. A. (2010). Role of fiber in cardiovascular diseases: A review. *Comprehensive reviews in food science and food safety, 9*(2), 240-258.

39. Anderson, J. W., Randles, K. M., Kendall, C. W., & Jenkins, D. J. (2004). Carbohydrate and fiber recommendations for individuals with diabetes: a quantitative assessment and meta-analysis of the evidence. *Journal of the American College of Nutrition, 23*(1), 5-17.

40. Mottet, C., & Michetti, P. (2005). Probiotics: wanted dead or alive. *Digestive and liver disease, 37*(1), 3-6.

41. Panahi, S., & Tremblay, A. (2016). The potential role of yogurt in weight management and prevention of type 2 diabetes. *Journal of the American College of Nutrition, 35*(8), 717-731.

42. Everard, A., & Cani, P. D. (2014). Gut microbiota and GLP-1. *Reviews in endocrine and metabolic disorders, 15*, 189-196.

43. Jayasinghe, T. N., Chiavaroli, V., Holland, D. J., Cutfield, W. S., & O'Sullivan, J. M. (2016). The new era of treatment for obesity and metabolic disorders: evidence and expectations for gut microbiome transplantation. *Frontiers in cellular and infection microbiology, 6*, 15.

44. Joglar, J. A., Chung, M. K., Armbruster, A. L., Benjamin, E. J., Chyou, J. Y., Cronin, E. M., ... & Van Wagoner, D. R. (2024). 2023 ACC/AHA/ACCP/HRS guideline for the diagnosis and management of atrial fibrillation: a report of the American College of Cardiology/American Heart Association Joint Committee on Clinical Practice Guidelines. *Circulation, 149*(1), e1-e156.

45. Sorli, C., Shin-ichi, H., & Tsoukas, G. (2016). Brand Name: Ozempic. *Diabetes, 375*(19), 1834-1844.

46. Chowdhury, Z. (2019). Mounjaro (Tirzepatide): Dual-Targeted Treatment for Type 2 Diabetes. *Yerevanian, A. and AA Soukas, Metformin: mechanisms in human obesity and weight loss. Current obesity reports, 8*, 156-164.

47. Haddad, F., Dokmak, G., Bader, M., & Karaman, R. (2023). A comprehensive review on weight loss associated with anti-diabetic medications. *Life, 13*(4), 1012.

48. Reinhild Haerig, T., Krause, D., Klaassen-Mielke, R., Rudolf, H., Trampisch, H. J., & Thuermann, P. (2023). Potentially inappropriate medication including drug-drug interaction and the risk of frequent falling, hospital admission, and death in older adults-results of a large cohort study (getABI). *Frontiers in Pharmacology, 14*, 1062290.

49. Nackers, L. M., Ross, K. M., & Perri, M. G. (2010). The association between rate of initial weight loss and long-term success in obesity treatment: does slow and steady win the race?. *International journal of behavioral medicine*, *17*, 161-167.

Exercise: The holy grail of health
By: Asim Syed MD, Kyair Smith MD, Jonathan Kahan MD

What you need to know:

1. Exercise is the greatest medicine available. The ability to exercise is more important than any other health factor and is the most important action you can take to improve your health.
2. Our goal is to improve health span, which we use VO2 Max as a surrogate for. Training this way breaks down into weight lifting/resistance training and cardio. Cardio further breaks down into base (zone 2) training and high intensity interval training at a ratio of 75/25.
3. All the specifics are less important than consistency. If you exercise regularly with effort, the rest makes very little difference, you will see vast improvements in your life and health.

What is our goal?

Our goal with exercise is to improve your health span, which is the length of time that a person is healthy, not just "alive". We are not training for a specific sport. Note that there are certain conditions where this plan will need to be modified, check with your doctor first.

How can I measure this?

We use VO2 Max as a surrogate for exercise capacity and health span. VO2 Max is the maximum rate of oxygen your body can use during exercise measured in milliliters of oxygen per kilogram of body weight per minute (mL/kg/min)[27]. Your body uses oxygen to create ATP (adenosine triphosphate) which is the energy molecule of all life processes. A higher VO2 Max means that you are able to handle more activities that require oxygen.

Why care about VO2 Max?

The people with the highest VO2 Max are also the people who live the longest and live with the best quality of life. In a study done of over 100,000 patients, VO2 Max was directly and inversely correlated with all-cause mortality.[12] This amounted to a 80%(!!!) reduction in all-cause mortality between the top 2% and bottom 25% of patients (elite vs low: adjusted hazard ratio [HR], 0.20; 95% CI, 0.16-0.24; $P < .001$).[12] Note this effect was more than smokers vs. nonsmokers. This is the number one metric that you have control over that can drastically affect your health span.

How to Measure VO2 Max?

The gold standard approach is to measure using a CPET (cardiopulmonary exercise test). This is where you run on a treadmill with a closed mask system. However, the smart watches are fairly accurate and can track your VO2 Max overtime. We recommend purchasing one (see social for other reasons) in order to follow this important metric. Another way to test is the Cooper test, where you record the maximum distance you are able to cover on a track/treadmill over 12 minutes (do your best!). Then use the formula VO2max = (35.97 x miles) - 11.29 and compare to your age/sex chart below.

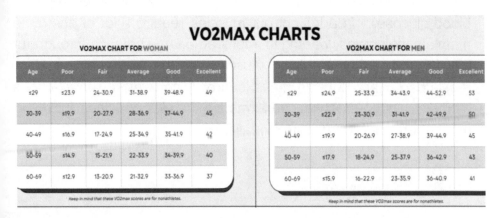

VO2MAX CHARTS

VO2MAX CHART FOR WOMAN

Age	Poor	Fair	Average	Good	Excellent
≤29	≤23.9	24-30.9	31-38.9	39-48.9	49
30-39	≤19.9	20-27.9	28-36.9	37-44.9	45
40-49	≤16.9	17-24.9	25-34.9	35-41.9	42
50-59	≤14.9	15-21.9	22-33.9	34-39.9	40
60-69	≤12.9	13-20.9	21-32.9	33-36.9	37

Keep in mind that these VO2max scores are for nonathletes.

VO2MAX CHART FOR MEN

Age	Poor	Fair	Average	Good	Excellent
≤29	≤24.9	25-33.9	34-43.9	44-52.9	53
30-39	≤22.9	23-30.9	31-41.9	42-49.9	50
40-49	≤19.9	20-26.9	27-38.9	39-44.9	45
50-59	≤17.9	18-24.9	25-37.9	36-42.9	43
60-69	≤15.9	16-22.9	23-35.9	36-40.9	41

Keep in mind that these VO2max scores are for nonathletes.

Figure 1: VO2 max chart for different genders and age.[26]

Who has the highest VO2 Max?

The people with the highest VO2 Max are endurance athletes, eg. cross country skiers, marathon runners, cyclists.[28] We will copy their training in order to maximize our VO2 Max and therefore our health span. Note also there are two ways based on the equation to improve your VO2 Max: either improve your oxygen utilization efficiency or lose weight.

How do they train?

The best endurance athletes in the world train in the following way: A. Weightlifting/resistance training with a mixture of B. 75% base (Zone 2) cardio and C. 25% HIIT training (High Intensity Interval Training).[31] These will be explored in depth below.

A. Weightlifting

Why should I weight lift/perform resistance training (RT)?

Resistance training (RT) can approximately reduce all-cause mortality by 15% and lower risk of CVD by 17% when compared with those who report no RT.[11] It reduces blood pressure and improves lipid profiles, as well as enhances our insulin sensitivity (muscles are sinks for sugar and are the main way we regulate blood glucose). In addition, our muscles require a lot of energy to maintain their mass, leading to improved energy balance throughout the day (other than the liver, muscles are the main way our body regulates sugar). Muscle mass is directly correlated with all-cause mortality, independence, performance in all capacities including mental, and cardiovascular mortality.[13]

Isn't weightlifting dangerous?

Weightlifting is safe.[14] The following activities are more dangerous from risk of injury than weightlifting.

Sports Injury Rates (Hamill 1994)

Sport	Injuries (per 100 hours)
Soccer (school age)	6.20
UK Rugby	1.92
USA Basketball	0.03
UK Cross Country	0.37
Squash	0.10
US Football	0.10
Badminton	0.05
USA Gymnastics	0.044
USA Powerlifting	0.0027
USA Volleyball	0.0013
USA Tennis	0.001
Weight Training	0.0035 (85,733 hrs)
Weightlifting	0.0017 (168,551 hrs)

Figure 2: Injuries seen in different exercises per 100 hours [14]

How many times a week should I weight lift/perform resistance training?

You should aim to target each muscle group twice per week.[11] Some exercises such as deadlifts target about 80% of your muscles, whereas a calf raise may target only one. Therefore, compound exercises (bench press, squats, deadlifts etc) are more efficient as they target multiple muscle groups at the same time. These can be performed effectively and safely with machines or with barbells/dumbbells. Kettlebells are also safe however maybe more advanced than traditional weightlifting. You will obtain 90% of weight lifting benefits by just showing up consistently and putting in more effort than reading a newspaper. You do not need fancy gyms or personal trainers, basic gyms are as cheap as $10 a month, have all the equipment you need and have free personal trainers to show you how to use it.

How should I warm up?

In general, a warmup for weightlifting can be minimal. We recommend just doing one set of 12 reps of lighter weights (see below), then another set of 6 reps of lighter weights than normal to warm up for the first exercise. After that you should train normally.[29]

How much weight should I use?

The rule of thumb is to start low and go slow. You should feel tension or stretch of the muscles during the exercise, a possible slight burning sensation (i.e. the lactic acid and other anaerobic metabolites), the "pump" of the muscle (water following increased blood flow) and a weakness/cramping sensation at the end. These are signs that the weight you are using is appropriate and that you are getting a good workout. It is important to note that less weight leads to less injury. Significant joint pain is bad, but you may experience some. Machines that only allow you to do one exercise are a great way to start. Most gyms will also offer free personal trainers who can show you how to begin weightlifting.

Panel A Resistance Training Prescription Components

RT Intensity	Percent of 1-RM	Number of Reps	Frequency per week	Muscle Adaptation	Population
Low Intensity	<40% 1-RM	15-20 reps	≥ 2 days/week	Endurance	High risk patients
Moderate Intensity	40-60% 1-RM	8-12 reps	≥ 2 days/week	Strength and endurance	General Population
High Intensity	>80% 1-RM	1-6 reps	≥ 2 days/week	Strength	Healthy adults looking to optimize strength

Figure 3. METS indicates metabolic equivalents of task; 1-RM, 1-repetition maximum; and RT, resistance training.[11]

How many sets/repetitions should I use?

Repetitions are the quantities of a specific movement you do, such as 10 biceps curls. Sets are the number of "blocks" of repetitions you do with resting in between e.g. 3 sets of 10 biceps curls. There is no difference between 5-20 repetitions per exercise or 1-6 sets. In general, the higher the repetitions the less weight per repetition you will use (leading to less injury, although this risk is low already), and the higher the number of sets the less likely you are to have good form at the end of those sets. Weight loads that permit 8-12 repetitions are ideal for building both muscle mass and muscle endurance. "For healthy adults, regimens of 8 to 10 different exercises involving major muscle groups, each exercise performed in 1 to 3 sets of moderate intensity loads that permits 8 to 12 repetitions per set to volitional fatigue, ≥2 times per week, is effective for achieving muscular and cardiovascular benefits."[11] These exercises should be targeted to major muscle groups. Note also that thinking of a mantra such as "blank" in between alternating reps makes the time go faster and swearing while lifting has been shown to increase strength[32]!

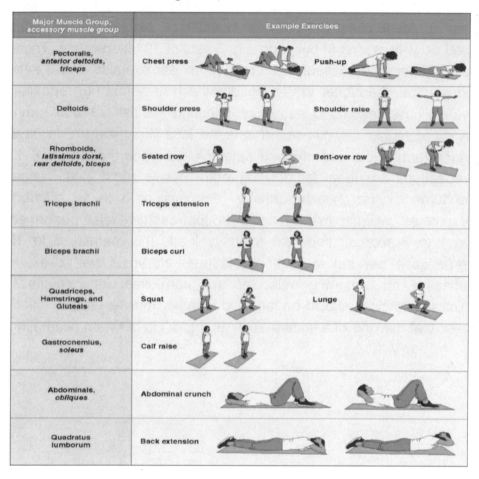

Major Muscle Group, accessory muscle group	Example Exercises			
Pectoralis, anterior deltoids, triceps	Chest press		Push-up	
Deltoids	Shoulder press		Shoulder raise	
Rhomboids, latissimus dorsi, rear deltoids, biceps	Seated row		Bent-over row	
Triceps brachii	Triceps extension			
Biceps brachii	Biceps curl			
Quadriceps, Hamstrings, and Gluteals	Squat		Lunge	
Gastrocnemius, soleus	Calf raise			
Abdominals, obliques	Abdominal crunch			
Quadratus lumborum	Back extension			

Figure 4: Exercises targeting major muscle groups[11]. Deadlifts, pull ups and rows are missing from this figure for back exercises. These can be looked up online and should be incorporated into the above.

How long to rest between sets?

This will vary depending on the exercise, for example you may need to rest several minutes between squat sets while resting only a few seconds between calf raises. In general your pulse should be under 100 bpm (ie. not tachycardic or short of breath) and your muscles (including smaller muscles used for stabilization) should not feel fatigued.[15] This is another great reason to buy a smart watch or a heart rate monitor. A good strategy given the above is to do leg workouts last or exercises that leave you with a fast heart rate or short of breath.

Does it matter total body vs. upper/lower split etc?

In general it does not matter whether you do total body workouts, or upper body one day and lower body the next etc. The order of the workout should be pre planned however and should make sense eg. not doing 3 bicep exercises in a row. Also writing down the exercises, sets, reps and weights is a great way to track progress and to see where you are having issues. Think critically, increase weight slowly over time once you are comfortable with the set/rep burden and are not experiencing the signs of growth as above. Consistency is key.

B. Cardio: base training (Zone 2) and High Intensity Interval Training

How much cardio should I get a week?

The real answer is however much is possible that fits your lifestyle (there is no upper limit to cardio). The minimum that is recommended is from the American Heart Association to prevent CVD is 30 minutes, 5 times a week to reach at least 150 minutes per week of moderate exercise (base training aka zone 2), or 25 minutes, 3 times a week to reach at least 75 minutes per week of vigorous activity (HIIT). We will see below why combining both types is best. For those who want to lower the risk for heart attack and stroke, 40 minutes of moderate to vigorous intensity aerobic activity, 3 or 4 times a week, is recommended.[1] Aerobic exercise has favorable effects on lipid metabolism, cardiac remodeling, post-MI heart failure, insulin resistance, and endothelial function all of which contribute to the favorable effects on cardiovascular fitness and decrease the risk of developing CVD and may even decrease CVD progression.[1,2]

How do I know when to take a rest day?

Persistent soreness, especially in the same muscle groups for 48 to 72 hours, decline in exercise performance, feeling fatigued despite a good night's rest, poor sleep, feeling mildly sick, and irritability or mood changes are all signs that you may need to take a recovery day. However, rest days can also be active, including things like yoga, dynamic stretching, walking etc.

What are the heart rate zones?

Heart rate zones are based on a percentage of your maximum heart rate. There are five zones.

Zone	Also known as	Intensity level	% of max heart rate	Fuel source
1	Warm up or recovery	Moderate to low	50-60	Fat
2	**Aerobic, endurance**	**Moderate**	**60-70**	**Fat**
3	Tempo, threshold, cardio, moderate.	Moderate to high	70-80	Fat, carbs and protein
4	Lactate threshold, redline, hard.	High	80-90	Carbs and protein
5	**Anaerobic, V02 max, peak, maximum.**	**Very High**	**90-100**	**Carbs and proteins**

Table 1: Zone training description, definition and fuel source[9]

Maximum heart rate is calculated using the formula 220-Age. For example, a person who is 40 years old would have a max heart rate of 220-40=180.[8,10]

What is base training aka zone 2 training?

Base training (zone 2) is considered the "fat burning zone". In reality, it is the threshold exercise level of which your body is using aerobic (oxygen) metabolism. Where else have we heard that? It is the definition of VO2 Max! Base training is the base of a triangle where the area is VO2 Max. This is achieved by increasing the body's ability to oxidize free fatty acids (FFA) which causes them to become energy in the form of ATP rather than becoming triglycerides or entering muscle cells to impair glucose tolerance. Additionally, they increase the density of mitochondria in cells as well, which are the energy producing power houses for our bodies.

How do I tell I am in my base zone aka fat burning zone?

The most accurate way is to measure your lactic acid thresholds using multiple finger prick tests, however this is not recommended or ideal for most people. The best next way to tell is that it is the level of cardio where you can carry on a conversation but that the conversation is difficult (but not impossible). This is going to be about 60-70% of your maximum predicted heart rate (= 220 - your age).[9,10] Smartwatches can detect it as well and have zones calibrated for each activity.

What is High Intensity Interval Training (HIIT)?

There is no standard definition for what HIIT training is. Basically, it is a period of near maximum exercise intensity followed by a period of rest or submaximal intensity. HIIT training improves the quality of mitochondria and increases our aerobic threshold as well.[17] Additionally, it is an extremely efficient way of exercising, meaning you can get a lot of work done in a short amount of time. Furthermore, many people find it more enjoyable than going at a slow steady pace for an extended period of time. There are multiple variations of HIIT including Tabata (2:1 intervals of high/low intensity), sprint intervals (near max for a short duration [seconds] in a 1:1 with recovery, repeated multiple times), EMOM (one minute on, one minute off etc.).[18-20] Note it takes time for the heart rate to ramp up to near maximum intensity. Therefore, in classic HIIT, if you look at studies, it was more near maximum intensity for 2-5 minutes! (not seconds) followed by some sort of similar duration of recovery. The classic Norwegian 4x4 of high to low intensity is the best studied where you do 4 min of 85-95% of max heart rate then 3-4 min of recovery like jogging or walking then repeat 4 times with a 10 min warm up and cool down.[21] HIIT training on a mitochondrial level improves the efficiency, and function of fatty acid oxidation as well, leading to improved VO2 max, an afterburn of increased energy utilization and increases the height of our VO2 Max triangle.

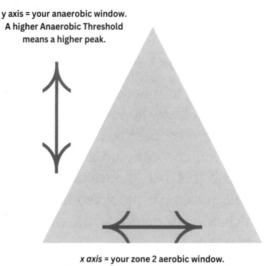

Figure 5- Relationship between anaerobic and aerobic threshold[30]

What ratio of base to HIIT Training should we aim for?

Generally, when we follow what long distance swimmers, cyclists, marathon runners and cross-country skiers are doing, they are training at approximately 75-80% base training and 20-25% HIIT training.[31] This way increases our mitochondrial density (with base training) while increasing efficiency and function (HIIT). This is to maximize the benefits of our VO2 Max triangle and to improve our health span, while minimizing risk of fatigue and injury.[31]

Other than VO2 Max, How does exercise affect my body?

Studies show that a sedentary lifestyle, characterized by consistently low levels of physical activity, is now recognized as a leading contributor to poor cardiovascular health and predisposes patients to the development of cardiovascular disease. In fact, according to the Global Burden of Disease Study, a lack of physical activity can be attributed to almost 10% of premature death worldwide![22] Conversely, regular exercise and increased physical activity, even low levels, are associated with widespread health benefits and a significantly lower CVD risk. Increasing physical activity showed a reduction in all-cause mortality and may modestly increase life expectancy, an effect which is strongly linked to a decline in the risk of developing cardiovascular and respiratory diseases.[23] Physical activity can improve insulin sensitivity, improve dyslipidemia, normalize elevated blood pressure, and improve overall health in many ways.[6] Even in people with coronary artery disease, an increase in regular physical activity can improve VO_2 max and, at high doses (~2,200 kcal burned/week), promote regression of atherosclerotic lesions. There is evidence that high levels of non HDL-C which comprises LDL-C, IDL-C, VLDL-C and lipoprotein a (Lpa) have been associated with increased cardiovascular disease. A combination of aerobic and resistance exercise can help lower non HDL-C and hence reduce CAD risk. [4,5]

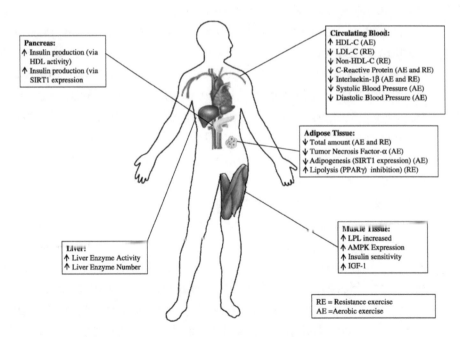

Figure 6- Physiological effects of exercise on the body [8]

What about Sauna? I have heard it is similar to moderate intensity exercise.

Beyond the relaxing benefits of saunas, new evidence suggests that sauna bathing has several cardiovascular benefits, which include reduction in the risk of high blood pressure, cardiovascular disease (CVD), stroke, neurocognitive diseases; respiratory illnesses; mortality; skin conditions; as well as pain in conditions such as rheumatic diseases and headache. The protocols however are tough, in that you need at least 20 minutes of sauna per session, at least 4 days a week, at a temperature of 80-100 degrees Celsius (176-212 F).[3] Note at this time infrared (IR) saunas are unable to reach these temperatures. Also note a hot bath/jacuzzi where the clavicle is able to be submerged may have similar benefits. Similarly to exercise, sauna can lead to a reduction in blood pressure, improvement in endothelial function, reduction in oxidative stress and inflammation, beneficial modulation of the autonomic nervous system, improved lipid profile and arterial compliance, and cause improvement in the cardiorespiratory system.[3] Therefore, sauna bathing may be a safer alternative for patients who are unable to do moderate physical activity. Increased frequency and duration of sauna bathing is associated with decreased risk of sudden cardiac death (SCD), fatal coronary heart disease and CVD, and all-cause mortality. Additionally, heat shock proteins are created which may be beneficial in cellular repair. The one caveat is that most of this data comes from Finland, where Sauna is a way of life. The French Paradox (where red wine was associated with longevity secondary to extensive use in French culture and not because of the wine itself) has not been ruled out here. A second caveat is that there is an opportunity cost, where saunas are not as prevalent in the US, and some people may prefer to exercise regularly instead of enduring the heat. However, we find the evidence regarding sauna use and cardiovascular outcomes compelling, and would suggest if you have access to one, that you should consider incorporating the protocols into your exercise regime.

References

1. Tian D, Meng J. Exercise for Prevention and Relief of Cardiovascular Disease: Prognoses, Mechanisms, and Approaches. *Oxid Med Cell Longev*. 2019;2019:3756750. Published 2019 Apr 9. doi:10.1155/2019/3756750
2. Schroeder EC, Franke WD, Sharp RL, Lee DC. Comparative effectiveness of aerobic, resistance, and combined training on cardiovascular disease risk factors: A randomized controlled trial. *PLoS One*. 2019;14(1):e0210292. Published 2019 Jan 7. doi:10.1371/journal.pone.0210292
3. Laukkanen JA, Laukkanen T, Kunutsor SK. Cardiovascular and Other Health Benefits of Sauna Bathing: A Review of the Evidence. *Mayo Clin Proc*. 2018;93(8):1111-1121. doi:10.1016/j.mayocp.2018.04.008
4. Leon AS, Sanchez OA. Response of blood lipids to exercise training alone or combined with dietary intervention. *Med Sci Sports Exerc*. 2001;33(6 Suppl):S502-S529. doi:10.1097/00005768-200106001-00021
5. Nystoriak MA, Bhatnagar A. Cardiovascular Effects and Benefits of Exercise. *Front Cardiovasc Med*. 2018;5:135. Published 2018 Sep 28. doi:10.3389/fcvm.2018.00135
6. Lobelo F, Rohm Young D, Sallis R, et al. Routine Assessment and Promotion of Physical Activity in Healthcare Settings: A Scientific Statement From the American Heart Association. *Circulation*. 2018;137(18):e495-e522. doi:10.1161/CIR.0000000000000559
7. Saint-Maurice PF, Troiano RP, Berrigan D, Kraus WE, Matthews CE. Volume of Light Versus Moderate-to-Vigorous Physical Activity: Similar Benefits for All-Cause Mortality? [published correction appears in J Am Heart Assoc. 2018 Dec 4;7(23):e03714]. *J Am Heart Assoc*. 2018;7(7):e008815. Published 2018 Apr 2. doi:10.1161/JAHA.118.008815
8. Current Sports Medicine Reports. 13(4):253-259, July/August 2014. - Figure 2
9. Exercise Heart Rate Zones Explained. Cleveland Clinic Health Essentials. Accessed May 7, 2024
11. Paluch AE, Boyer WR, Franklin BA, Laddu D, Lobelo F, Lee DC, McDermott MM, Swift DL, Webel AR, Lane A; American Heart Association Council on Lifestyle and Cardiometabolic Health; Council on Arteriosclerosis, Thrombosis and Vascular Biology; Council on Clinical Cardiology; Council on Cardiovascular and Stroke Nursing; Council on Epidemiology and Prevention; Council on Peripheral Vascular Disease. Resistance Exercise Training in Individuals With and Without Cardiovascular Disease: 2023 Update: A Scientific Statement From the American Heart Association. Circulation. 2023; 149:e217-e231. doi:10.1161/CIR.0000000000001189
12. Mandsager K, Harb S, Cremer P, Phelan D, Nissen SE, Jaber W. Association of Cardiorespiratory Fitness With Long-term Mortality Among Adults Undergoing Exercise Treadmill Testing. *JAMA Netw Open*. 2018;1(6):e183605. doi:10.1001/jamanetworkopen.2018.3605
13. Zhou Y, Hellberg M, Svensson P, Höglund P, Clyne N. Low Skeletal Muscle Mass Index and All-Cause Mortality Risk in Adults: A Systematic Review and Meta-Analysis of Prospective Cohort Studies. J Clin Endocrinol Metab. 2023;108(3). doi:10.1371/0268745
14. Hamill, R P Relative safety of weightlifting and weight training. J. Strength and CondoRes. 8(1):53-57.1994
15. de Salles BF, Simão R, Miranda F, Novaes Jda S, Lemos A, Willardson JM. Rest interval between sets in strength training. Sports Med. 2009;39(9):765-77. doi: 10.2165/11315230-000000000-00000. PMID: 19691365.
16. Thompson WR. Worldwide Survey of Fitness Trends for 2021, ACSM's Health & Fitness Journal. 1/2 2021. Volume 25; Issue 1: 10-19.

17. MacInnis MJ, Gibala MJ. Physiological adaptations to interval training and the role of exercise intensity. *J Physiol*. 2017;595(9):2915-2930. doi:10.1113/JP273196

18. Tabata I, Nishimura K, Kouzaki M, et al. Effects of moderate-intensity endurance and high-intensity intermittent training on anaerobic capacity and VO2max. *Med Sci Sports Exerc*. 1996;28(10):1327-1330. doi:10.1097/00005768-199610000-00018

19. Weston M, Taylor KL, Batterham AM, Hopkins WG. Effects of low-volume high-intensity interval training (HIT) on fitness in adults: a meta-analysis of controlled and non-controlled trials. *Sports Med*. 2014;44(7):1005-1017. doi:10.1007/s40279-014-0180-z

20. O'Malley, C., & Mazzetti, S. (2018). The effects of high-intensity interval training vs. steady state training on aerobic and anaerobic capacity. Journal of Exercise Physiology Online, 21(5), 102-112.

21. Acala JJ, Roche-Willis D, Astorino TA. Characterizing the Heart Rate Response to the 4 × 4 Interval Exercise Protocol. *Int J Environ Res Public Health*. 2020;17(14):5103. Published 2020 Jul 15. doi:10.3390/ijerph17145103.

22. Murray CJL. The Global Burden of Disease Study at 30 years. Nat Med. 2022;28:2019-2026. doi:10.1038/s41591-022-01735-0

23. Grandes G, García-Alvarez A, Ansorena M, et al. Any increment in physical activity reduces mortality risk of physically inactive patients: prospective cohort study in primary care. *Br J Gen Pract*. 2022;73(726):e52-e58. Published 2022 Dec 21. doi:10.3399/BJGP.2022.0118

24. VO2max Charts by Age, Gender & Sport. Inscyd. https://inscyd.com/article/vo2max-charts-by-age-gender-sport/. Accessed May 10, 2024.

25. Bundy M, Leaver A. Chapter 1 - Training and conditioning. In: Bundy M, Leaver A, eds. A Guide to Sports and Injury Management. Churchill Livingstone; 2010:1-9. doi:10.1016/B978-0-443-06813-3.00004-1.

26. Bassett DR Jr, Howley ET. Limiting factors for maximum oxygen uptake and determinants of endurance performance. Med Sci Sports Exerc. 2000;32(1):70.

27. Ribeiro B, Pereira A, Neves PP, et al. The Role of Specific Warm-up during Bench Press and Squat Exercises: A Novel Approach. *Int J Environ Res Public Health*. 2020;17(18):6882. Published 2020 Sep 22. doi:10.3390/ijerph17186882

28. Building Our Metabolic Triangle. Envision Endeavor. https://www.envisionendeavor.com/p/building-our-metabolic-triangle. Accessed May 11, 2024.

29. Casado A, González-Mohíno F, González-Ravé JM, Foster C. Training Periodization, Methods, Intensity Distribution, and Volume in Highly Trained and Elite Distance Runners: A Systematic Review. *Int J Sports Physiol Perform*. 2022;17(6):820-833. doi:10.1123/ijspp.2021-0435

30. Stephens, R., Dowber, H., Barrie, A., Almeida, S., & Atkins, K. (2023). Effect of swearing on strength: Disinhibition as a potential mediator. *Quarterly journal of experimental psychology (2006)*, 76(2), 305–318. https://doi.org/10.1177/17470218221082657

Sleep and Its Impact on Cardiovascular Health
By: Kyair Smith MD, Benjamin Ravaee MD, Jonathan Kahan MD

What you need to know

- Sleep is part of the cornerstone of cardiovascular health. If you have poor sleep, it is very difficult to be healthy from a cardiovascular standpoint.
- Medications, substances, and supplements rarely work for sleep and have side effects that destroy sleep architecture, diminishing the health benefits of sleep.
- Today our sleep is worse than ever before. A lot of people struggle with sleep, it's ok! There are good techniques to help with sleep. If they don't work, a sleep expert is available as well.

Why do we need sleep?

Sleep is a necessary physiological process essential for overall health and well-being. Beyond its role in rest and restoration, emerging research has highlighted the intricate connections between sleep patterns and cardiovascular health. In this exploration, we delve into the multifaceted relationship between sleep and cardiovascular disease (CVD) while exploring the effects of sleep on cardiovascular fitness.

How does sleep work?

There are two main biological processes that regulate our sleep; the first one being circadian rhythm where the environment inputs onto our internal clock, and the second being sleep homeostasis and pressure regulated by adenosine levels. Our internal biological clock, also known as the suprachiasmatic nucleus (SCN), functions to coordinate our bodies' activity levels to the rising and setting of the sun using hormones and the autonomic nervous system. To generate and coordinate automatic processes such as heart rate, wakefulness, and hormone levels, the SCN requires repeated metabolic cues from environmental factors such as light exposure, sleep, activity, and feeding.[1] On the other hand, adenosine and its receptors are postulated to play a role in sleep pressure and intensity. Adenosine is a consequence of cellular metabolism and is produced from the breakdown of ATP, a cellular energy source. Thus, the longer we are awake and active, the more adenosine accumulates in the areas of our brain related to arousal.[2] The accumulation of adenosine translates to increased sleep pressure which allows you to fall asleep earlier and more deeply.

What are sleep stages?

There are five stages of sleep: awake, N1, N2, N3, and Rapid Eye Movement (REM). Approximately 75% of sleep is spent in the non-REM (NREM) stages (N1-N3), with the majority spent in the N2 stage. A typical night's sleep consists of 4 to 5 sleep cycles (each approximately 90-120 minutes long), with the progression of sleep stages in the following order: N1, N2, N3, N2, REM. The N1 stage is the lightest form of sleep, it occurs during the first 1-5 minutes of falling asleep, and is the shortest phase of the sleep cycle. The N2 stage is a deeper sleep, characterized by specific brain waves known as sleep spindles and/or K complexes. These distinctive patterns are only found in N2 sleep and are thought to be caused by the intense neuronal firing that occurs during memory consolidation.[3]

The N3 stage, also known as the slow wave stage, is the deepest form of sleep and is the time when rejuvenating processes such as tissue repair and regrowth, bone and muscle formation, and the immune system resets occur. Last is the Rapid Eye Movement (REM) stage. During REM sleep, the body remains paralyzed, but the muscles of the eyes and the diaphragm are not, thus the characteristic rapid eye movement that can be observed. Interestingly, the amount of REM we experience decreases as we age, with infants having the highest levels of REM. This leads to the hypothesis that REM sleep plays an important role in memory consolidation, emotional development and motor learning.[4]

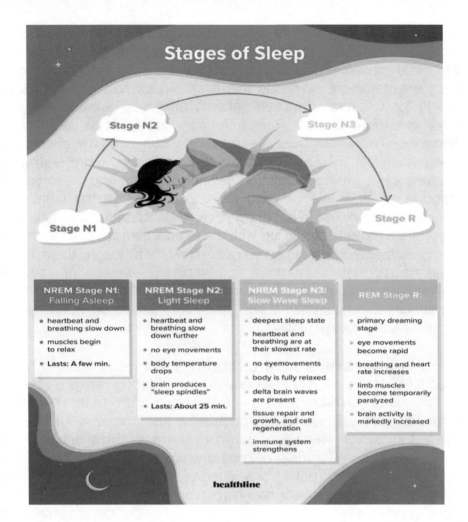

Figure 1. Stages of Sleep[4]

How does sleep chronotype affect sleep?

Sleep chronotypes are defined as an individuals' natural proclivity to sleep during a certain time of day[5]. Most experts agree on 2 major categories of sleep chronotypes- earlier or later chronotypes with some reports of intermediate types. The earlier chronotypes are what many would refer to as a "morning person" or "early bird". These people prefer to wake up earlier, experience peak physical and mental activity closer to awakening, around 10am-noon, and go to sleep earlier as well. Conversely, the later chronotypes are characteristically known as "night owls," persons who prefer to wake up later around 10-11am, peak activity around 3-6pm and fall asleep later in the night.

When our sleeping habits are in misalignment with our internal biological time clock, this is referred to as circadian misalignment. If this misalignment is due to social obligations such as school, work, even entertainment purposes this is known as social jet lag (SJL) due to the difference in sleep patterns observed between working days and free days.[6] Research has proven that our sleep chronotype may affect our sleep quality, with negative effects on sleep, such as increased difficulty falling asleep, more nighttime awakenings, greater caffeine consumption, and decreased amounts of REM sleep being more prominent in the night owl groups. Similarly, studies show that later chronotypes typically experience more social jet lag with the effects being insomnia, mood changes, fatigue, and difficulty concentrating; although, there have been no reported differences in objective measures of daytime alertness and cognitive functioning.[6] Chronotype can therefore predict circadian disruption, and as such, affect sleep-wake cycles and potentially sleep quality.

The conclusion that evening chronotypes are more likely to have circadian misalignment and increased sleep debt gives us a clue as to why later chronotypes are associated with more negative cardiovascular effects. More specifically, just one hour of SJL or sleep debt, which has been shown to be more prevalent in night owls, increases the risk of cardiovascular disease by 11%.[5] Contributing to this point, one observational study showed that individuals who sleep later had higher body mass index (BMI), ate more calories after 8:00 PM, and had less healthy diets overall.[7] In addition, individuals with a preference for later bedtimes were more likely to be obese, have diabetes and/or hypertension, further indicating the role sleep chronotypes may play in cardiovascular disease.[7]

With this in mind, those who identify as later chronotypes could make attempts to alter their chronotype in order to avoid the negative health effects associated with circadian misalignments, although this may be easier said than done. Since chronotype is mainly dependent on non-modifiable factors such as age, gender, genes, and geographical location, studies that attempted to alter chronotype have only been successful in changing the median sleep time for at most two hours by making changes in behavioral and environmental input.[8] This can be done by setting your alarm 2 hours earlier, eating a high protein first meal, getting outside early (direct sunlight, no glass filter!) and exercising earlier, as well as going to bed earlier by 2-3 hours.

If you are unsure which type you are, you can look up the MEQ test, which is a 20 questions that will tell you which chronotype you are.

How much sleep should I get?

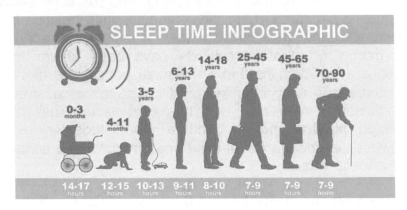

Figure 2. How much sleep do we need according to age[9].

The duration of sleep plays a crucial role in cardiovascular health. The National Sleep Foundation recommends 8 hours of sleep a night to maintain optimal health in adults. Unfortunately, studies show that the average duration of sleep in Western societies has decreased from 9 hours in 1910 to less than 7 hours today.[9] And even more concerning, people who do shift work, defined as any job that operates outside of the typical 8am-5pm (including parents of young children!), often report getting 5 hours of sleep or less. This is roughly 15 million Americans; including health care providers, factory workers, firefighters, bartenders, food service workers, and many more that fall into this category. Epidemiological studies have consistently demonstrated a U-shaped relationship between sleep duration and the incidence of coronary heart disease (CHD), with both short and long sleep durations associated with an increased risk.[9]

Short sleep durations, defined as less than five hours per night, have been linked to hypertension, atherosclerosis, and other cardiovascular conditions due to their detrimental effects on metabolic and inflammatory pathways.[10] Sleeping less than 5 hours a night could lead to hypertension through elevated sympathetic

111

nervous system activity, increased cortisol (the stress hormone), and increased catecholamines (fight or flight response), causing elevated blood pressure (BP) the next day.[11,12] Similarly, chronic sleep deprivation leads to structural adaptations by the cardiovascular system to adjust to continued elevated BPs, such as arterial and ventricular hypertrophy and remodeling which can also contribute to worsening cardiovascular function.[13] Additionally, chronic short sleep durations could also contribute to hypertension by disrupting circadian rhythmicity and autonomic balance by way of decreased metabolic activity due to altered sensory input. Furthermore, hypertensive subjects have been shown to have reductions of >50% in the 3 main neuronal populations of the SCN in comparison to normal subjects.[10] Conversely, excessively long sleep durations may also add to cardiovascular risk through decreased physical activity, and a more sedentary lifestyle, suggesting the importance of achieving optimal sleep duration for cardiovascular health.

How Does Sleep Quality Impact Cardiovascular Health?

Beyond sleep duration, the quality of sleep significantly influences cardiovascular outcomes. Poor sleep quality, characterized by frequent awakenings, disturbances in sleep architecture, and sleep disorders such as sleep apnea, contribute to the development and progression of cardiovascular disease. Additionally, studies have shown that acute sleep deprivation during the first part of the night causes the physiologic drop in blood pressure and heart rate to be blunted during the hours of sleep deprivation. This causes increased BP readings the following day which is supported by an increase in urinary excretion of norepinephrine and epinephrine observed during the sleep-deprivation night.[12]

Elevated plasma concentrations of C-reactive protein (CRP) are indicative of systemic (chronic) inflammation and are used as a marker for cardiovascular health and fitness. In a study conducted by Meier-Ewert et al. where they measured levels of high-sensitivity C-reactive protein (hs-CRP) in healthy adults who stayed awake for 88 continuous hours; the hs-CRP concentrations and systolic BP increased during the period of sleep deprivation, which further demonstrates a relationship with sleep deprivation and cardiovascular inflammation.[14]

How does sleep apnea affect sleep?

Obstructive sleep apnea (OSA), in particular, is associated with increased sympathetic nervous system activity, oxidative stress, and endothelial dysfunction, all of which promote cardiovascular pathology and increase the risk of adverse cardiovascular events.[15,16] These changes may be related to patients' lifestyle, meaning the daytime somnolence caused by sleep apnea may predispose individuals to a lack of physical activity, to consume more calories and consequently gain weight. The increase in weight, more specifically increased deposition of fat in the upper respiratory system causes further narrowing of the airways which worsens the sleep apnea, causing a vicious cycle.[17]

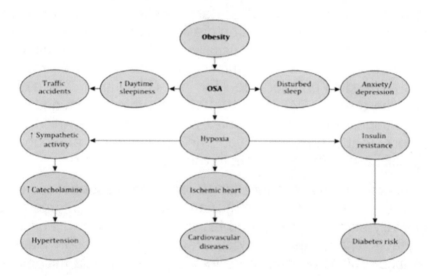

Figure 3. The Effects of OSA as it Relates to Cardiovascular Disease and its Risk Factors[18]

How does caffeine affect sleep?

Coffee/Caffeine has been shown to have beneficial health effects, such as reducing the risk for some types of cancer, decreasing the chances of developing diabetes, and lowering the risk for heart disease and stroke to name a few (note coffee specifically is America's main way of obtaining antioxidants and over 90% of people worldwide are coffee drinkers)[20]. Research shows that these benefits of coffee are attributable to both the caffeine and antioxidant/anti-inflammatory properties. Caffeine has persistently shown to lower the risk of type 2 diabetes (antioxidant effect), as well as improved lipid profiles and cardiovascular health.[20] Caffeine is an adenosine-receptor blocker, it functions to oppose the homeostatic properties of adenosine on sleep. Therefore, caffeine causes increased alertness and arousal by blocking the natural effects of adenosine and delaying sleep homeostasis and decreasing sleep pressure.[2] Caffeine is found in a number of foods and beverages, such as coffee, tea, dark chocolate, medications and energy drinks, with an average cup of coffee containing around 95 milligrams of caffeine.[20] Decaffeinated coffee, produced by extracting caffeine from coffee beans, contains significantly less caffeine, typically ranging from 2 to 5 milligrams per 8-ounce cup but delivers the same aroma and flavor as a regular cup of coffee.

It is important to note that there are several ways to decaffeinate coffee, with the water or carbon dioxide methods being the safest. The effects of caffeine can usually be felt within 30 minutes of consumption; however, the effects can last anywhere from 2-10 hours depending on tolerance (The half (T½) life of caffeine is 5-6 hours, the quarter (T¼) life is 10-12 hours), metabolism and genetic factors (highly variable CYP450/AHR gene clearance which we can test for). That means that if you drink coffee in the afternoon, you may still have caffeine present in your system at night!

We recommend no caffeine after 12 pm at the latest because of this. Caffeine in the afternoon/night can lead to sleep fragmentation, especially stage 3-4 sleep and blunting of N1 sleep. Habitual use can lead to upregulated adenosine receptors in the brain, leading to tolerance. Taking occasional caffeine breaks can help mitigate this. Of note energy drinks are not safe, as they contain very high levels of caffeine (in addition to sugars and other harmful additives) and can be consumed very quickly (why the army has banned their use as it can lead to arrhythmias which may be fatal).

How does alcohol affect sleep?

Although many report using alcohol to help fall asleep (due to its sedative effects), the metabolites of alcohol can significantly disrupt sleep throughout the night as they are continuously metabolized in the liver. A standard drink contains approximately 14 grams of ethanol. This will reach peak blood levels in about an hour, but it will take approximately 25 hours to be cleared from the body entirely. However, the effects of alcohol depend on the amount consumed, the rate of metabolism, the speed of consumption, BMI, gender and several other factors. Alcohol increases N3 sleep at the beginning of the night, but it suppresses REM sleep, which causes significant sleep fragmentation and awakenings during the latter half of the night, leading to overall nonrestorative sleep.[21] Additionally, chronic alcohol consumption and/or alcohol use disorder has been shown to disrupt the circadian rhythm and sleep homeostasis, leading to worsened symptoms of sleep apnea, insomnia and vivid dreams in others.[21] These effects can lead to worsened withdrawal symptoms and increased chances of relapse in those with alcohol dependence.

How does nicotine affect sleep?

Smoking is one of the biggest modifiable risk factors of cardiovascular disease. We know it has negative effects on the body in general but how does it affect our sleep more specifically? When we smoke the effects of nicotine are felt almost immediately, but may take up to 30 minutes for most, and the effects of nicotine wear off within 2-3 hours of consumption. The effects of nicotine consumption are difficulty falling asleep, increased nighttime awakenings, and decreased restorative slow wave sleep and REM sleep causing increased daytime sleepiness.[22] These symptoms are more pronounced in individuals who smoke later in the day or closer to bedtime, likely due to nicotine withdrawal occurring while the person is asleep. Additionally, nicotine withdrawal causes increased depression and worsened sleep disturbances which could contribute to smoking relapse, further worsening the sleep disturbances associated with nicotine.[22]

What about marijuana's effect on sleep?

Marijuana (and the active ingredient THC) interact with endocannabinoid receptors in the brain to affect sleep. The effects of THC on sleep are dose dependent. THC binds to these receptors and increases adenosine (thereby increasing sleep pressure) as well as enhancing GABA, which is the primary inhibitory neurotransmitter. This can help users fall asleep quicker and increase the amount of slow wave sleep, however this can also lead to dependence on the drug to fall asleep.[23] As tolerance develops over time to all drugs, this can lead to higher and higher dosing requirements. Additionally, long term use and higher dose

115

requirements alters sleep architecture by increasing slow wave sleep but suppressing REM sleep (which is why withdrawal leads to vivid dreaming) and diminished sleep quality.[23] While short term benefits may exist with marijuana use in sleep, long term changes in sleep architecture and dependence suggests cautious use at best.

How do sleep aids affect sleep?

For those who have issues with sleeping, sleep aides such as Benadryl and Ambien are commonly used to achieve a better night's rest. Benadryl, a common over-the-counter antihistamine containing diphenhydramine, is sometimes used off-label as a sleep aid due to its sedating effects and easy availability. However, its use as a sleep aid is generally not recommended as it can lead to several adverse effects, including daytime drowsiness, dizziness, cognitive impairment, and a heightened risk of falls, particularly in older adults. Additionally, studies have linked the chronic use of diphenhydramine-containing sleep aids with an increased risk of mortality, especially in older individuals.[24] Specifically, in regards to cardiovascular health diphenhydramine has been known to increase heart rate and in higher doses can cause arrhythmias (irregular heartbeats), cardiac arrest, and even death.[22] Similarly, prescription sleep aids like Ambien (zolpidem) have also been associated with potential risks including dependency, rebound insomnia once discontinued, impaired driving, and an increased risk of falls, accidents and cardiovascular events. More specifically, a Japanese study showed that use of sleeping pills increases the risk of cardiovascular events in heart failure patients by 8-fold.[25] As such, healthcare professionals generally advise against the long-term use of these medications for managing sleep disturbances, emphasizing the importance of non-pharmacological approaches and the careful consideration of risks versus benefits when using sleep aids.

How does melatonin affect sleep?

Melatonin is a hormone that is produced in the pineal gland, and has important effects on the circadian rhythm, as an antioxidant and in possible immunomodulation and gut microbiome interaction. Light inhibits melatonin production while darkness increases its release. Even indoor light can inhibit this release. Melatonin only helps speed up the onset of sleep, it has nothing to do with sleep quantity or quality overall. In 2022 1.6 billion dollars of Melatonin OTC was sold in the US, including to children. Analysis of this melatonin shows up to 450% higher dosing than is advertised on the bottle, as well as significant variability in dosing between batches from the same company.[26] Furthermore, melatonin only increases the speed to sleep by a few minutes (7 minutes in some meta-analysis).[27] Given lack of regulation, efficacy and long term chronic use safety data, we do not recommend melatonin except for jet lag and short use cases (4-8 weeks).

How does my sleep environment affect sleep?

The ideal room temperature is 63-68°F. As melatonin levels rise during sleep, our body's core temperature inversely decreases, therefore, colder room temperatures have been shown to cause increased melatonin release which promotes increased sleep.[28] Conversely, studies have shown that increased sleeping temperatures can dysregulate our REM sleep, and cause sleep disruption, whereas cooler sleeping environments have been shown to cause increased N3 sleep, the most restorative stage of the sleep cycle.[29] Similarly, it is important to minimize distractions in our sleep environment like loud noises and bright lights as these factors can all disrupt sleep and cause nighttime awakenings.

While natural light exposure during the day is beneficial for regulating the circadian rhythm, exposure to artificial light sources in the evening, particularly blue-rich light, can interfere with the body's internal clock and disrupt sleep and melatonin production. Therefore, reducing exposure to screens and artificial light sources that are high in blue-light, especially in the hours leading up to bedtime, may promote better sleep hygiene and overall sleep health. Many have jumped on the trend of blue light blockers, most commonly in the form of screen protectors or glasses. Studies suggest that wearing blue light blockers in the evening does improve sleep quality and increase melatonin levels (although results are mixed).[30] Moreover, the engagement with stimulating content on social media platforms can further exacerbate sleep problems by increasing cognitive arousal/awakeness and delaying the onset of sleep (regardless of blue light). Therefore, it is important to reduce screen time 1-2 hours before bed regardless of blue light blocking on not. Furthermore, sleeping in a cold, quiet room will promote a restful night of rest.

How does exercise affect sleep?

As we are discussing sleep as it relates to cardiovascular health it is important to consider exercise, one of the biggest promoters of cardiovascular health and fitness. Exercise can have a significant impact on sleep quality and duration, with numerous studies highlighting its positive effects on various aspects of sleep. Regular physical activity, especially aerobic exercise, has been shown to reduce the time it takes to fall asleep.[31] Increased activity earlier in the day helps to regulate our circadian clock making us more alert and energized during the day. Furthermore, it promotes the onset of sleep at night, increases sleep depth due to increased tiredness, and decreases the number of nighttime awakenings. Also, exercise can help relieve stress and boost mood, which may improve sleep as mental health issues are a major contributor to insomnia and sleeping difficulties.[31]

While the exact mechanisms underlying this relationship are not fully understood, it is believed that the physiological and psychological benefits of exercise contribute to improved sleep continuity and overall sleep duration. Overall, incorporating regular exercise into one's daily routine can lead to numerous benefits for sleep health, including faster sleep onset, improved sleep quality, reduced sleep disturbances, and enhanced overall sleep duration. However, it's essential to avoid vigorous exercise too close to bedtime, as it may have stimulating effects that could interfere with the ability to fall asleep. Therefore, exercise is recommended for earlier in the day, more specifically, mornings for those with circadian disruption.

How does sauna/heat prior to sleep affect sleep?

Similar to exercise, the use of sauna may also promote better sleep through stress reduction, muscle relief, and increased release of endorphins (the hormones involved in increased mood). Heat from Saunas, hot showers or baths initially may delay sleep (see above). However, the rapid decrease in body temperature after exiting is a potent sleep inducer, much the same way as a cold environment is conducive to sleep. Aim for a hot shower/heat exposure 1-2 hours prior to bed.

How does sleep affect eating habits?

Lack of sleep can significantly impact our eating habits and metabolism, leading to changes in calorie intake and levels of important hormones such as leptin and ghrelin. When we don't get enough sleep, our body's internal regulation of appetite and hunger can become disrupted. This disruption often leads to an increase in appetite and cravings for high-calorie, carbohydrate-rich foods. Studies have shown that sleep-deprived individuals tend to consume more calories, particularly from snacks and comfort foods, compared to those who get adequate sleep.[32] Leptin, a hormone produced by fat cells, helps the brain to understand when we are full. Similarly, the hormone ghrelin, produced by the stomach, signals to the brain when we are hungry and promotes food intake and hunger.

A lack of sleep disrupts the delicate balance of these two hormones, leading to decreased levels of leptin and increased ghrelin; causing increased feeding and less satiety.[33] Furthermore, if this pattern continues, they may also develop leptin resistance which is implicated in obesity. Inadequate sleep can also affect the body's ability to metabolize carbohydrates, leading to insulin resistance and potentially increasing the risk of weight gain and metabolic disorders over time.[34] Overall, the interplay between sleep, eating habits, and hormonal regulation underscores the importance of prioritizing sufficient sleep for maintaining a healthy weight and metabolism.

What are the biological mechanisms underlying sleep-related cardiovascular risk?

Numerous biological mechanisms underlie the relationship between sleep and cardiovascular health. Chronic sleep deprivation disrupts neuroendocrine regulation, leading to dysregulation of cortisol, leptin, and ghrelin levels, thereby promoting insulin resistance and obesity, both of which are established risk factors for cardiovascular disease. Additionally, alterations in autonomic nervous system activity, including increased sympathetic tone and decreased

119

parasympathetic activity, contribute to adverse cardiovascular outcomes by affecting heart rate variability, vascular tone, and endothelial function.

In conclusion, sleep exerts profound effects on cardiovascular health, influencing blood pressure regulation, endothelial function, metabolic homeostasis, and overall cardiovascular fitness. Sleep plays a crucial role in modulating blood pressure, hormone levels, body temperature, and restoration of our bodies. Recognizing the intricate interplay between sleep patterns and cardiovascular physiology is essential for implementing effective strategies for cardiovascular disease prevention and management. By prioritizing sleep hygiene, addressing sleep disorders, promoting regular physical activity, and optimizing treatment of cardiovascular risk factors, healthcare professionals can optimize cardiovascular health and improve patient outcomes in both clinical and community settings.

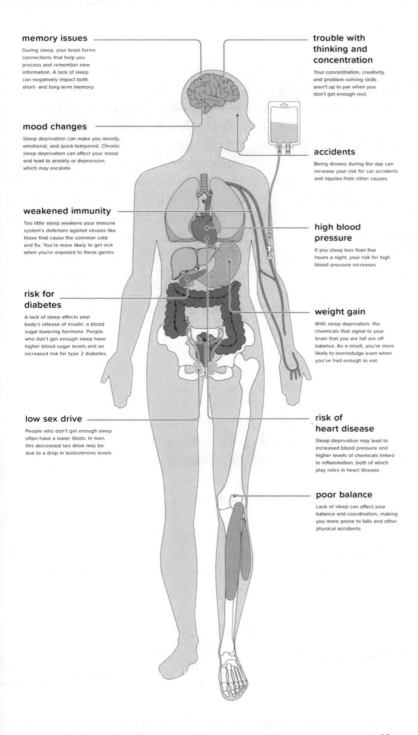

memory issues

During sleep, your brain forms connections that help you process and remember new information. A lack of sleep can negatively impact both short- and long-term memory.

mood changes

Sleep deprivation can make you moody, emotional, and quick-tempered. Chronic sleep deprivation can affect your mood and lead to anxiety or depression, which may escalate.

weakened immunity

Too little sleep weakens your immune system's defenses against viruses like those that cause the common cold and flu. You're more likely to get sick when you're exposed to these germs.

risk for diabetes

A lack of sleep affects your body's release of insulin, a blood sugar-lowering hormone. People who don't get enough sleep have higher blood sugar levels and an increased risk for type 2 diabetes.

low sex drive

People who don't get enough sleep often have a lower libido. In men, this decreased sex drive may be due to a drop in testosterone levels.

trouble with thinking and concentration

Your concentration, creativity, and problem-solving skills aren't up to par when you don't get enough rest.

accidents

Being drowsy during the day can increase your risk for car accidents and injuries from other causes.

high blood pressure

If you sleep less than five hours a night, your risk for high blood pressure increases.

weight gain

With sleep deprivation, the chemicals that signal to your brain that you are full are off balance. As a result, you're more likely to overindulge even when you've had enough to eat.

risk of heart disease

Sleep deprivation may lead to increased blood pressure and higher levels of chemicals linked to inflammation, both of which play roles in heart disease.

poor balance

Lack of sleep can affect your balance and coordination, making you more prone to falls and other physical accidents.

Figure 4. The 11 effects of sleep deprivation on your body[35]

What is insomnia?

Everyone has one or many bad sleep nights for a variety of reasons and this is not insomnia. Insomnia can be divided into sleep onset insomnia and sleep maintenance insomnia. Sleep onset insomnia is defined as taking at least 30 minutes to fall asleep, or 30 minutes to go back to sleep, at least 3 nights a week for 3 months in a row[37]. On the other hand, sleep maintenance insomnia (middle insomnia) is defined as nighttime awakenings at least twice a week for one month that at least moderately impacts your life, but without difficulty falling asleep initially. These two definitions are opposed to sleep deprivation, where you have the ability to fall and stay asleep but don't have the opportunity (eg. young kids, shift work, etc). Polysomnography (sleep studies) do not aid in diagnosis, the best way to diagnose insomnia is with a test called the insomnia severity index and by keeping a sleep diary for at least 2 weeks.

What causes insomnia?

The 3P model of insomnia states that 33% of insomnia is predisposition (hereditary), 33% is due to precipitating factors eg. social factors such as stress, fighting, rumination, conflict etc, and 33% is attributed to perpetuating factors such as eating or drinking the wrong things (alcohol, caffeine, nicotine etc).[36]

How do I treat/avoid insomnia (or if I just have trouble sleeping)?

- Start the day off with natural bright light exposure. Natural light is preferred but any light input onto your eyes will help alert the body that it is morning. (Note that glass blocks the photons for this light.)
- It is better to exercise and eat larger meals earlier in the day, as this helps regulate the circadian rhythm. Specifically, high-intensity exercise leads to increased adenosine levels which will increase sleep pressure and make it easier to fall asleep later.
- Avoid long naps during the day since napping will decrease the adenosine levels in your brain, leading to decreased sleep pressure and difficulty falling asleep later.

- Napping in increments of 20 minutes has been shown to have the most beneficial effects.
- Note it is normal to feel tired at the 1-4 pm time frame. This is part of a normal circadian rhythm. There is a theory that we are biphasic sleepers, meaning we were meant to sleep for two periods. We recommend following this chapter's advice and the midafternoon slump should be kept to a minimum.

- Avoid caffeine, nicotine and alcohol at least 4 hours before bed since these substances can make it harder to fall asleep, stay asleep and may disrupt your sleep cycle. If you are sensitive to these substances, you will need to just stop using them.
- Decrease bright light exposure at least 4 hours before sleeping to help regulate your circadian rhythm. Try light dimmers (dim to half light), blue light filters/glasses, and reduced screen time to achieve these effects.
- Avoid large meals 2-3 hours before bedtime as they can cause circadian disruption as well as gas, bloating, reflux may interrupt or make it difficult to sleep. Additionally, avoid drinking beverages 1 hour before bed, to decrease nighttime awakenings due to thirst or the need for urination.
  - The 3,2,1 rule works well here, 3 hours before bed is the last meal, 2 hours is the last electronic use, 1 hour is the last drink (nonalcoholic).
- Try to limit screens (computers, cell phones and television, etc.) while in bed, the bed should only be used for sleep and intimacy. This helps the brain to associate the bed with sleep and increased sleep onset.
- Melatonin supplementation may help in those with circadian disruption, although its effects are not robust. It should not be used long term.
- Keep the room temperature between 63-68°F, keep the room as dark as possible and minimize noise throughout the night for an ideal sleep environment.
- Do not stay in bed awake for more than 20-30 minutes; if sleeping is difficult, try getting out of the bed and doing a relaxing activity for 10 minutes, then returning to the bed.
- If you stay in bed awake for a long time (poor sleep efficiency), then compress sleep time (i.e. shift bedtime from 12 AM to 2 am to force sleep pressure). Once you are

sleeping 100% of those hours gradually move the bedtime back up.

- eg. in bed from 12 am - 8 am but only sleeping for 5 hours? Move sleep time up to 2 am-8 am (efficiency improves to 100%, therefore now getting 6 hours of sleep), then gradually move bedtime earlier.

• Try to maintain a regular sleep, light/dark, mealtime and exercise schedule. Keeping these activities as routine as possible entrains your biological rhythms for maximal alertness during the day and maximal sleepiness during the night.

• Try to get between 7-10 hours of sleep every night, with the requirement changing depending on your age.

• If sleep becomes continuously difficult (see insomnia definitions above), it may be time to see a sleep specialist about a potential sleep disorder. They are fantastic and can offer many treatment options beyond this book such as cognitive behavioral therapy.

References

1. Zou, H., Zhou, H., Yan, R., Yao, Z., & Lu, Q. (2022). Chronotype, circadian rhythm, and psychiatric disorders: Recent evidence and potential mechanisms. *Frontiers in Neuroscience, 16*. https://doi.org/10.3389/fnins.2022.811771
2. Reichert CF, Deboer T, Landolt HP. Adenosine, caffeine, and sleep-wake regulation: state of the science and perspectives. *J Sleep Res.* 2022;31(4):e13597. doi:10.1111/jsr.13597
3. Patel, A. K., Reddy, V., & Araujo, J. F. (2022, September 7). *Physiology, Sleep Stages.* PubMed; StatPearls Publishing. https://www.ncbi.nlm.nih.gov/books/NBK526132/#:~:text=Sleep%20occurs%20in%20five%20stages
4. *The Stages of Sleep: What Happens During Each.* (2020, June 18). Healthline. https://www.healthline.com/health/healthy-sleep/stages-of-sleep#tips-for-sleep
5. HARFMANN, B. D., SWALVE, N., MITRZYK, J., & MONTOYE, A. H. K. (2020). Effect of Chronotype on Sleep Quality in a Laboratory Setting. *International Journal of Exercise Science, 13*(3), 1283–1294. https://www.ncbi.nlm.nih.gov/pmc/articles/PMC7523902/
6. Caliandro, R., Streng, A. A., van Kerkhof, L. W. M., van der Horst, G. T. J., & Chaves, I. (2021). Social Jetlag and Related Risks for Human Health: A Timely Review. *Nutrients, 13*(12), 4543. https://doi.org/10.3390/nu13124543
7. Baron KG, Reid KJ, Kern AS, Zee PC. Role of sleep timing in caloric intake and BMI. *Obesity (Silver Spring).* 2011;19(7):1374-1381. doi:10.1038/oby.2011.100
8. *Can You Change Your Chronotype (And How?) – Fit Sapiens.* (n.d.). Fit Sapiens. Retrieved April 18, 2024, from https://fitsapiens.org/how-you-can-change-your-chronotype/#:~:text=and%20%E2%80%9Ctype.%E2%80%9D-
9. *Tired all the time? Here's a formula for the perfect night's sleep.* (n.d.). World Economic Forum. https://www.weforum.org/agenda/2022/05/ideal-hours-sleep-study/
10. Pickering, T. G. (2006). Could Hypertension Be a Consequence of the 24/7 Society? The Effects of Sleep Deprivation and Shift Work. *The Journal of Clinical Hypertension, 8*(11), 819–822. https://doi.org/10.1111/j.1524-6175.2006.05126.x
11. Nagai, M., Hoshide, S., & Kario, K. (2010). Sleep Duration as a Risk Factor for Cardiovascular Disease- a Review of the Recent Literature. *Current Cardiology Reviews, 6*(1), 54–61. https://doi.org/10.2174/157340310790231635

12. Gangwisch, J. E., Heymsfield, S. B., Boden-Albala, B., Buijs, R. M., Kreier, F., Pickering, T. G., Rundle, A. G., Zammit, G. K., & Malaspina, D. (2006). Short Sleep Duration as a Risk Factor for Hypertension. *Hypertension*, *47*(5), 833–839. https://doi.org/10.1161/01.hyp.0000217362.34748.e0

13. Paola Lusardi, Annalisa Zoppi, Paola Preti, Rosa Maria Pesce, Elena Piazza, Roberto Fogari, Effects of insufficient sleep on blood pressure in hypertensive patients: A 24-h study, American Journal of Hypertension, Volume 12, Issue 1, January 1999, Pages 63-68, https://doi.org/10.1016/S0895-7061(98)00200-3

14. Matsubayashi, H., Nagai, M., Dote, K., Turana, Y., Siddique, S., Chia, Y., Chen, C., Cheng, H., Van Minh, H., Verma, N., Chin Tay, J., Wee Teo, B., & Kario, K. (2020). Long sleep duration and cardiovascular disease: Associations with arterial stiffness and blood pressure variability. *The Journal of Clinical Hypertension*, *23*(3), 496–503. https://doi.org/10.1111/jch.14163

15. Meier-Ewert, H. K., Ridker, P. M., Rifai, N., Regan, M. M., Price, N. J., Dinges, D. F., & Mullington, J. M. (2004). Effect of sleep loss on C-Reactive protein, an inflammatory marker of cardiovascular risk. *Journal of the American College of Cardiology*, *43*(4), 678–683. https://doi.org/10.1016/j.jacc.2003.07.050

16. LEUNG, RICHARD S. T., & DOUGLAS BRADLEY, T. (2001). Sleep Apnea and Cardiovascular Disease. *American Journal of Respiratory and Critical Care Medicine*, *164*(12), 2147–2165. https://doi.org/10.1164/ajrccm.164.12.2107045

17. Wolk, R., Shamsuzzaman, A. S. M., & Somers, V. K. (2003). Obesity, Sleep Apnea, and Hypertension. *Hypertension*, *42*(6), 1067–1074. https://doi.org/10.1161/01.hyp.0000101686.98973.a3

18. Tai JE, Phillips CL, Yee BJ, Grunstein RR. (2024) Obstructive sleep apnoea in obesity: A review. *Clinical Obesity*. 2024;e12651. https://doi.org/10.1111/cob.12651

19. Jehan S, Zizi F, Pandi-Perumal SR, et al. (2017) Obstructive sleep apnea and obesity: implications for public health. *Sleep Medicine Disorders International Journal*;1(4):93-99. DOI: 10.15406/smdij.2017.01.00019

20. Harvard School of Public Health. (2019, January 8). *Coffee*. The Nutrition Source. https://www.hsph.harvard.edu/nutritionsource/food-features/coffee/

21. Colrain, I. M., Nicholas, C. L., & Baker, F. C. (2014). Alcohol and the sleeping brain. *Handbook of Clinical Neurology*, *125*, 415–431. https://doi.org/10.1016/b978-0-444-62619-6.00024-0

22. Jaehne, A., Loessl, B., Bárkai, Z., Riemann, D., & Hornyak, M. (2009). Effects of nicotine on sleep during consumption, withdrawal and replacement therapy. *Sleep Medicine Reviews*, *13*(5), 363–377. https://doi.org/10.1016/j.smrv.2008.12.003

23. Vaillancourt R, Gallagher S, Cameron JD, Dhalla R. (2022) Cannabis use in patients with insomnia and sleep disorders: Retrospective chart review. *Can Pharm J (Ott)*. 2022;155(3):175-180. doi:10.1177/17151635221089617

24. Kim, Y.-H., Kim, H.-B., Kim, D.-H., Kim, J.-Y., & Shin, H.-Y. (2018). Use of hypnotics and the risk of or mortality from heart disease: a meta-analysis of observational studies. *The Korean Journal of Internal Medicine*, *33*(4), 727–736. https://doi.org/10.3904/kjim.2016.282

25. European Society of Cardiology (ESC). Sleeping pills increase cardiovascular events in heart failure patients, study finds. ScienceDaily. Published 2014 May 17. Accessed May 2, 2024. Available from: <www.sciencedaily.com/releases/2014/05/140517085835.htm>.

26. Grigg-Damberger MM, Ianakieva D. Poor Quality Control of Over-the-Counter Melatonin: What They Say Is Often Not What You Get. J Clin Sleep Med. 2017;13(2):163-165. doi:10.5664/jcsm.6434

27. Ferracioli-Oda E, Qawasmi A, Bloch MH. Meta-analysis: melatonin for the treatment of primary sleep disorders. PLoS One. 2013;8(5):e63773. doi:10.1371/journal.pone.0063773

28. Burgess HJ, Sletten T, Savic N, Gilbert SS, Dawson D. Effects of bright light and melatonin on sleep propensity, temperature, and cardiac activity at night. J Appl Physiol (1985). 2001;91(3):1214-1222. doi:10.1152/jappl.2001.91.3.1214

29. Good Sleep Recipe. Medicine.yale.edu. Accessed May 2, 2024. Available from: https://medicine.yale.edu/internal-medicine/pulmonary/news/national-sleep-week/good-sleep-recipe/#:~:text=In%20essence%2C%20the%20longer%20you.

30. Wood B, Rea MS, Plitnick B, Figueiro MG. Light level and duration of exposure determine the impact of self-luminous tablets on melatonin suppression. *Appl Ergon*. 2013;44(2):237-240. doi:10.1016/j.apergo.2012.07.008

31. Alnawwar MA, Alraddadi MI, Algethmi RA, Salem GA, Salem MA, Alharbi AA. The Effect of Physical Activity on Sleep Quality and Sleep Disorder: A Systematic Review. Cureus. 2023;15(8):e43595. doi:10.7759/cureus.43595

32. St-Onge, M.-P., Roberts, A. L., Chen, J., Kelleman, M., O'Keeffe, M., RoyChoudhury, A., & Jones, P. J. (2011). Short sleep duration increases energy intakes but does not change energy expenditure in normal-weight individuals. The American Journal of Clinical Nutrition, 94(2), 410–416. doi:10.3945/ajcn.111.013904
33. Gomes S, Ramalhete C, Ferreira I, Bicho M, Valente A. Sleep Patterns, Eating Behavior and the Risk of Noncommunicable Diseases. *Nutrients*. 2023;15(11):2462. Published 2023 May 25. doi:10.3390/nu15112462
34. Spiegel, K., Knutson, K., Leproult, R., Tasali, E., & Cauter, E. V. (2005). Sleep loss: a novel risk factor for insulin resistance and Type 2 diabetes. *Journal of Applied Physiology*, 99(5), 2008–2019. https://doi.org/10.1152/japplphysiol.00660.2005
35. Watson, S., & Cherney, K. (2020, May 15). *11 Effects of Sleep Deprivation on Your Body*. Healthline; Healthline. https://www.healthline.com/health/sleep-deprivation/effects-on-body
36. Frontiersin.org. (2019). Perceived Social Support and Subjective Well-Being Among Chinese Adolescents: The Mediating Role of Emotional Intelligence. Frontiers in Psychology. Published 2019 Oct 29. Accessed May 2, 2024. Available from: https://www.frontiersin.org/journals/psychology/articles/10.3389/fpsyg.2019.02498/full.
37. Tian, C., Wei, Y., Xu, M., Liu, J., Tong, B., Ning, J., ... & Ge, L. (2024). The effects of exercise on insomnia disorders: An umbrella review and network meta-analysis. *Sleep Medicine*.

Social and Miscellaneous Topics
By: Jonathan Kahan MD

What you need to know

- The evidence for this section of the book is less certain, as social aspects of life are never in isolation and supplements/non cardiac pharmacology studies tend to be smaller, newer and less established. However, making some of these changes can have an outsized impact on your life and health.
- Cell phones, screens and social media are the "processed food" of social interaction and removing them from your life is excellent for your overall well-being. Find a purpose higher than yourself, get out in nature, and have real face to face interactions.

What about protein powder?

Protein powder comes in a variety of forms, the most beneficial version from a cardiovascular disease standpoint is whey protein from eggs/dairy. Whey is superior to plant protein powder as it contains a variety of amino acids not found in the plant form. The effects of protein powder have been shown to be beneficial in a variety of cardiovascular conditions including high blood pressure, type II diabetes, cholesterol, endothelial function, and even inflammation. Protein powders are absorbed rapidly, typically within 30-45 minutes. Note that you can only absorb 25-30 grams of protein per meal, and with whole food that absorption takes 3-4 hours[1]. Therefore, protein powders represent an excellent way to get to our recommendation of 1.5 grams of protein per kilogram of body weight daily.

Note that in healthy patients, the concern for kidney issues with a higher protein diet is minimal. Note also that if you have trouble obtaining this goal, you can take a scoop of protein powder in your fasting window to make it up, as this is more of a priority than the calories ingested from the protein itself. Lastly note that muscle is receptive to protein over 24 hours after exercise, and it is not crucial to consume a high protein meal immediately after exercise.

What about creatine?

Creatine is dosed typically at 5 grams/day and is available OTC. It is used by athletes to improve strength and high intensity exercises and may aid in recovery. There is limited evidence of improvement in conditions such as congestive heart failure (the heart is a muscle) and ischemic heart disease[2]. One concern is that it leads to water retention which may increase blood pressure. We recommend checking with your physician to see if creatine supplementation is the right option for you.

What about microplastics?

A very important study published in the New England Journal of Medicine in March of 2024 demonstrated the dangers of microplastics (tiny plastic particles <5 mm in diameter) from a CVD standpoint[3]. Three hundred patients had their carotid plaques removed surgically and examined for microplastics, which appear as jagged edges of debris with surrounding inflammation. Patients who had microplastics detected were at a significantly higher risk of heart attacks, strokes and all cause death (HR 4.53, 95% CI 2-10.27, p< 0.001). The main way that microplastics enter our bodies is by ingestion of food and liquid. Drinking water, both plastic bottled and tap, can contain significant amounts. We recommend installing a reverse osmosis filtration system or other filter systems to prevent ingestion and to avoid all liquids that are in plastic bottles (especially those stored on shelves)[4]. Note most fridge filters do not remove microplastics. Drinking exclusively from non-plastic containers should also be pursued. Note hot food or liquid can microscopically melt all plastics (regardless of type), and therefore avoid using plastic containers when food/liquid is hot. Paper coffee cups actually are lined with plastic to prevent spillage as are most coffee makers (especially pods). Shellfish accumulate more microplastic than any other food source. This is an area of ongoing research.

What about SGLT-2 Inhibitors?

Sodium-glucose cotransporter-2 (SGLT2) inhibitors are a class of medications that are mainly used in type 2 diabetes by preventing glucose reabsorption from the kidneys, resulting in excretion in the urine. SGLT2 inhibitors are showing a lot of promise in the arena of primary cardiovascular prevention[5]. They decrease the epicardial (visceral) fat around the heart (epicardial fat is associated with negative outcomes in cardiovascular longevity)[6]. In trials they have been shown to lower rates of cardiovascular death or hospitalizations secondary to congestive heart failure. While these studies were performed in diabetic patients, there are significant advances in studies for non-diabetic patients, warranting a closer look at SGLT-2 inhibitors as a mainstay of cardiovascular prevention in the future.

What about Vitamin C Supplementation?

Vitamin C has been shown to improve endothelial function (even at lower doses of 500 mg) and modest reduction in blood pressures (at higher doses of 2000 mg)[7]. Lastly, ascorbic acid (the most common vitamin C formulation) blood levels were shown to be inversely correlated with all-cause mortality and cardiovascular mortality. We recommend taking 500-1000 mg of vitamin C daily. Food sources are always best, in this case red bell peppers, citrus fruits, strawberries and broccoli. If you cannot obtain these there are OTC supplements.

What about vitamin D supplementation?

Vitamin D is the worst named vitamin of all the common ones. It is a steroid hormone involved in multiple processes and pathways in the body. Humans can produce vitamin D through sunlight (note there are increased cardiovascular events in winter and further from the equator), food (sardines/fatty fish are the best source) or by supplementation. It is also genetically determined. Vitamin 25-OH D deficiency is defined as < 20 ng/mL, insufficiency 20-40 ng/mL, optimal approx. 40-60 ng/mL and too high being >80 ng/mL, In the NHANES trial, 68% of white, 88% of Hispanic and 97% of black patients were deficient in Vitamin D[8,9]. Vitamin D mainly comes from sunlight exposure on skin, sardines, salmon, mackerel. OTC supplements are available and cheap. Dosing varies and we aim more to obtain optimal blood levels consistently. Note there is a prescription version of Vitamin D you will need to obtain if your blood levels are low enough (ask your physician). Vitamin D is involved in regulation of the renin-angiotensin system, which is one of the main regulators of blood pressure, and adequate vitamin D levels can lead to improved blood pressure[10]. It has anti-inflammatory effects (inflammation is a key driver of atherosclerosis aka plaque in the arteries) as well as calcium regulation which is key for cardiac function and vascular compliance. Lastly, while outside the scope of this book, the VITALS trial showed significant improvement in cancer all-cause mortality after one year latency in patients who had adequate vitamin D[11].

What about magnesium supplementation?

There are a multitude of magnesium supplements available, with magnesium chloride/glycinate (for premature extra ventricular contractions and cardiovascular health) and magnesium oxide (for gastrointestinal health) having the best absorption. The dose is 400 mg to 800 mg daily and is available OTC[12]. Magnesium helps stabilize heart rhythms, and high dietary magnesium was associated with lower cardiovascular mortality, congestive heart failure, blood pressure and stroke[13]. While magnesium can easily be measured in serum, with a goal level of 1.7-2.2 mEq/L, it is important to note that 99% of magnesium is sequestered in bone/cells, with serum levels only representing 1%. Therefore, occasionally testing red blood cell (RBC) magnesium levels, looking for deficiency symptoms and risk factors such as muscle cramping, arrhythmia, irritability, and gastrointestinal/kidney disorders and medication uses (antibiotics, diuretics etc.). Data on Magnesium threonate is mixed at this time, while it does cross the blood brain barrier, the trials in humans used a combination of supplements such as vitamin D[14,15]. This version of magnesium is classically used for sleep and to restore neurologic deficits.

What about homocysteine?

Homocysteine is an amino acid in blood that is elevated when patients are deficient in vitamin B12. A large proportion of the population have MTHFR gene mutations and are unable to absorb vitamin B12 in its native form[16]. This can be tested in blood and the treatment is to take methylated B12, which can be purchased OTC. In theory homocysteine may contribute to CVD by potentially damaging blood vessels, however studies at this time have shown a more limited role of homocysteine levels and cardiovascular disease[17].

What about meditation?

Meditation has been shown to improve blood pressure, heart rate variability (variation in time between heart beats, the higher the better), reduced stress/anxiety and inflammation and a 2017 meta-analysis showed it may reduce the risk of hypertension and stroke[18]. Various forms of meditation have been shown to help including mindfulness meditation, transcendental meditation, yoga etc. Most studies examined regular practice usually daily with 10-30 minutes a day. However, persistent meditation associated side effects run in the 10% range (we bet you didn't know there were any side effects)[19]! Most common side effects were anxiety, trauma re-experience and emotional instability, with childhood adversity increasing the risk of side effects. Hyperarousal and dissociation also occurred persistently at approximately a 10% rate. It is important to balance the benefits of meditation with potential side effects, especially if you have childhood traumas.

What about dental health?

Inflammation can occur in the gums and teeth, which can be detected on bloodwork and therefore in theory can lead to cardiovascular disease. In fact poor dentition has been shown to correlate with cardiovascular disease. However, treating isolated inflammation from the oral cavity has not shown as of yet to significant outcomes in terms of cardiovascular health. Regardless, oral health is essential for several reasons such as pain avoidance, being able to eat the foods you want, avoidance of dental procedures in the future, and overall lifestyle, health and wellbeing, especially as we age. Note also that children are having more dental procedures/braces over generations secondary to lack of chewing as a result of processed food[30]. Therefore, we recommend in addition to an unprocessed diet, avoid acidic drinks (also processed food), brush teeth twice daily for 2 minutes each, floss regularly and see your dentist!

What about mTOR inhibitors/longevity medications?

Are there substances that, when given to healthy individuals, expand lifespan beyond what would be normal? This is the area of longevity

131

medicine. The mammalian target of rapamycin (mTOR) is a signaling protein that is central to several key cell processes including growth and proliferation, nutrient sensing (via amino acids), growth factor sensing (like insulin), autophagy (programmed cell death) and lipid metabolism (for cell membranes)[20]. There are two mTOR inhibitors that are emerging in the literature as potential potent cardiovascular and longevity enhancers. The first is Quercetin which is OTC and found in fruits, vegetables, teas and red wine. Quercetin is a flavonoid that inhibits mTOR, is a potent antioxidant, improves blood sugar (enhances GLUT4 in muscle cells), increases nitric oxide (which reduces blood pressure), and enhances endothelial function. Typical doses are 500-1000 mg daily, and typically enhanced absorption with vitamin C or Bromelin. Multiple studies have shown benefit in a wide range of cardiovascular categories, albeit small and non randomized[21]. Rapamycin (aka sirolimus) was discovered as an antibiotic on Easter Island and is commonly used in immunosuppression for transplants. However, taking intermittent dosing (it is by prescription only), appears to inhibit mTOR complex 1 without affecting complex 2 (which carries most of the side effects)[22]. Rapamycin has been shown to enhance longevity in mouse models by up to 30% (when mice took in middle age). Rapamycin in humans has shown to improve immune function and chronic inflammation. As aging is the most common risk factor for all cardiovascular disease, it remains to be seen whether medications like mTOR inhibitors will play a role in cardiovascular disease prevention. At this time, it is unclear whether this class of supplement/medication will lead to improved cardiovascular outcomes, although the class appears promising and worth watching in the future. Note also at this time, NAD/NMN boosters have not shown significant longevity outcomes in mammals, though research is ongoing[23].

What about substances that increase nitric oxide?

Beetroot juice and phosphodiesterase-5 (PDE-5) inhibitors (sildenafil aka Viagra, tadalafil aka Cialisis) etc both increase nitric oxide concentration, which leads to vasodilation and significant drops in blood pressure. Furthermore, the PDE-5 inhibitors may improve endothelial function and enhance cardiac contractility. Indeed, studies have shown improvement in major adverse cardiovascular outcomes and all cause mortality in men with erectile dysfunction using PDE-5 inhibitors[30]. The downside is potential severe hypotension (low blood pressure), which may be fatal.

Further studies are needed, however this is another area of promising research in the field of primary prevention for cardiovascular health.

What about social media and cell phone use?

According to recent studies, the average person spends 2 hours and 23 minutes per day on social media and 4 hours and 39 minutes daily on cell phones in general[24]. This is an enormous quantity of time to spend on devices and on social media in particular. Social media in general is the processed food of interaction. It is empty of substance, specifically designed to manipulate you to feel anxious, isolated, addicted, depressed and sick[25]. Most of the time you are not even interacting with a real person but rather a bot, an influencer presenting a fake existence, or a known person showing only a small, highly curated, slice of their life. It disrupts sleep and negatively influences lifestyle choices such as inactivity, fear of missing out (FOMO), and substance use. Furthermore, users are sedentary and isolated throughout the use, which are factors significantly associated with increased risk of death from all causes and particularly cardiovascular causes[26]. Even the comments from people you know cannot be trusted, as the comments made would never occur in real life (both positive and negative). This goes for texting as well. Note that when mammals are isolated, they are easily manipulated into addictive, negative and repetitive behavior. News organizations take advantage of this hourly, showing only the worst of society and further causing harm. The giant opportunity cost of losing interaction and activity in the real world, in addition to the above, makes social media and cell phone use in general an extensive risk factor that negatively impacts users' health and wellbeing on multiple levels. Social media, given the above, is no longer the "town square" where people can get reliable information (it's currently podcasts and individual blogs where accurate information comes from). This line of technology has clearly made us weaker and less resilient/healthy. We recommend zero use of social media and news ingestion and a limited use of cell phones. While there may be positive aspects to social media use (like nicotine use is to mood), the negative aspects vastly outweigh the positive (like smoking is to cardiovascular health). Note we are not against technology per se, as many advances have helped people tremendously. As an example, we do advocate for smartwatches which can perform calls and texts and have health benefits such as tracking, positive motivation etc. However, when that technology causes such clear and obvious harms, it must be abandoned with the same speed and completeness as it was initiated. See next paragraph for further detail.

What about religion, marriage, having kids, being in nature and other real-world interactions?

Across the board and among most studies, being religious (regardless of which religion), being married and having kids, being in a natural environment and having actual social interactions in the real world is associated with significant improvements in cardiovascular health and longevity outcomes. Religious practice leads to improved social support (a stable community), provides a sense of purpose higher than oneself, offers stress reduction (prayer and meditation), healthier lifestyle practices etc. In the Nurses' Health Study, women who attended regular services had a 33% lower chance of death from cardiovascular causes[27]. Marriage and having children in meta-analyses resulted in moderate reductions in all-cause mortality and survival from coronary artery disease and congestive heart failure (surprisingly more so in men than women)[28]. Single and separated/divorced males had the poorest outcomes in terms of cardiovascular disease mortality and morbidity of any subgroup. Essentially, having a purpose higher than yourself (regardless of said purpose) appears to be beneficial from a cardiovascular standpoint. The World Health Organization lists air pollution from cities as a substantial contributor to cardiovascular disease[29]. Additionally, being in nature has been shown to have positive effects on the prevention of ischemic cardiomyopathy, reductions in blood pressure, and improved outlook on life. To tie all of the above together, it has been known for decades that real social interactions and social support mitigates cardiovascular stressors, reducing the risk of addiction, anxiety/depression, hypertension and limiting ischemic and non-ischemic cardiovascular disease risk, all while providing a purpose in life by focusing on something bigger than ourselves. We recommend a minimum of 4 hours and 39 minutes without a cell phone anywhere near you during your downtime, and a daily minimum of 2 hours and 23 minutes in real face to face human social interaction, in addition to being in nature and seeing the sun regularly. This is human technology and it works really well.

References

1. Schoenfeld, B. J., & Aragon, A. A. (2018). How much protein can the body use in a single meal for muscle-building? Implications for daily protein distribution. *Journal of the International Society of Sports Nutrition*, *15*, 1-6.

2. Balestrino, M. (2021). Role of creatine in the heart: Health and disease. *Nutrients*, *13*(4), 1215.

3. Marfella, R., Prattichizzo, F., Sardu, C., Fulgenzi, G., Graciotti, L., Spadoni, T., ... & Paolisso, G. (2024). Microplastics and nanoplastics in atheromas and cardiovascular events. *New England Journal of Medicine*, *390*(10), 900-910.

4. Mejjad, N., Laissaoui, A., Bouh, H. A., El Aouidi, S., Moumen, A., Azidane, H., & El Bouhaddioui, M. (2024). Analytical Review of Microplastics Occurrence in Bottled Water, Tap Water, and Wastewater Treatment Plants. In *E3S Web of Conferences* (Vol. 489, p. 06005). EDP Sciences.

5. Zelniker, T. A., Wiviott, S. D., Raz, I., Im, K., Goodrich, E. L., Bonaca, M. P., ... & Sabatine, M. S. (2019). SGLT2 inhibitors for primary and secondary prevention of cardiovascular and renal outcomes in type 2 diabetes: a systematic review and meta-analysis of cardiovascular outcome trials. *The Lancet*, *393*(10166), 31-39.

6. Masson, W., Lavalle-Cobo, A., & Nogueira, J. P. (2021). Effect of SGLT2-inhibitors on epicardial adipose tissue: a meta-analysis. *Cells*, *10*(8), 2150.

7. Morelli, M. B., Gambardella, J., Castellanos, V., Trimarco, V., & Santulli, G. (2020). Vitamin C and cardiovascular disease: an update. *Antioxidants*, *9*(12), 1227.

8. Linos, E., Keiser, E., Kanzler, M., Sainani, K. L., Lee, W., Vittinghoff, E., ... & Tang, J. Y. (2012). Sun protective behaviors and vitamin D levels in the US population: NHANES 2003–2006. *Cancer Causes & Control*, *23*, 133-140.

9. Zerwekh, J. E. (2008). Blood biomarkers of vitamin D status. *The American journal of clinical nutrition*, *87*(4), 1087S-1091S.

10. Norman, P. E., & Powell, J. T. (2014). Vitamin D and cardiovascular disease. *Circulation research*, *114*(2), 379-393.

11. Keaney, J. F., & Rosen, C. J. (2019). VITAL signs for dietary supplementation to prevent cancer and heart disease. *N Engl J Med*, *380*(1), 91-93.

12. Tangvoraphonkchai, K., & Davenport, A. (2018). Magnesium and cardiovascular disease. *Advances in chronic kidney disease*, *25*(3), 251-260.

13. Kolte, D., Vijayaraghavan, K., Khera, S., Sica, D. A., & Frishman, W. H. (2014). Role of magnesium in cardiovascular diseases. *Cardiology in review*, *22*(4), 182-192.

14. Ni, Y., Deng, F., Yu, S., Zhang, J., Zhang, X., Huang, D., & Zhou, H. (2023). A Randomized, Double-Blind, Placebo-Controlled Trial to Evaluate the Therapeutic Effect of Magnesium-L-Threonate Supplementation for Persistent Pain After Breast Cancer Surgery. *Breast Cancer: Targets and Therapy*, 495-504.

15. Zhang, C., Hu, Q., Li, S., Dai, F., Qian, W., Hewlings, S., ... & Wang, Y. (2022). A Magtein®, Magnesium L-Threonate,-Based Formula Improves Brain Cognitive Functions in Healthy Chinese Adults. *Nutrients*, *14*(24), 5235.

16. Marini, N. J., Gin, J., Ziegle, J., Keho, K. H., Ginzinger, D., Gilbert, D. A., & Rine, J. (2008). The prevalence of folate-remedial MTHFR enzyme variants in humans. *Proceedings of the National Academy of Sciences*, *105*(23), 8055-8060.

17. Ganguly, P., & Alam, S. F. (2015). Role of homocysteine in the development of cardiovascular disease. *Nutrition journal*, *14*, 1-10.

18. Shi, L., Zhang, D., Wang, L., Zhuang, J., Cook, R., & Chen, L. (2017). Meditation and blood pressure: a meta-analysis of randomized clinical trials. *Journal of hypertension*, *35*(4), 696-706.

19. Britton, W. B., Lindahl, J. R., Cooper, D. J., Canby, N. K., & Palitsky, R. (2021). Defining and measuring meditation-related adverse effects in mindfulness-based programs. *Clinical Psychological Science*, *9*(6), 1185-1204.

20. Jia, G., Aroor, A. R., Martinez-Lemus, L. A., & Sowers, J. R. (2014). Overnutrition, mTOR signaling, and cardiovascular diseases. *American Journal of Physiology-Regulatory, Integrative and Comparative Physiology, 307*(10), R1198-R1206.

21. Zhang, W., Zheng, Y., Yan, F., Dong, M., & Ren, Y. (2023). Research progress of quercetin in cardiovascular disease. *Frontiers in Cardiovascular Medicine, 10.*

22. Suda, M., Katsuumi, G., Tchkonia, T., Kirkland, J. L., & Minamino, T. (2024). Potential clinical implications of senotherapies for cardiovascular disease. *Circulation Journal, 88*(3), 277-284.

23. Norambuena-Soto, I., Deng, Y., Brenner, C., Lavandero, S., & Wang, Z. V. (2024). NAD in pathological cardiac remodeling: Metabolic regulation and beyond. *Biochimica et Biophysica Acta (BBA)-Molecular Basis of Disease*, 167038.

24. Howarth, Josh. "Time Spent Using Smartphones (2022 Statistics)." *Exploding Topics,* Exploding Topics, 9 Jan. 2023, explodingtopics.com/blog/smartphone-usage-stats.

25. Braghieri, L., Levy, R. E., & Makarin, A. (2022). Social media and mental health. *American Economic Review, 112*(11), 3660-3693.

26. Xia, N., & Li, H. (2018). Loneliness, social isolation, and cardiovascular health. *Antioxidants & redox signaling, 28*(9), 837-851.

27. Gillum, R. F., King, D. E., Obisesan, T. O., & Koenig, H. G. (2008). Frequency of attendance at religious services and mortality in a US national cohort. *Annals of epidemiology, 18*(2), 124-129.

28. Manfredini, R., De Giorgi, A., Tiseo, R., Boari, B., Cappadona, R., Salmi, R., ... & Fabbian, F. (2017). Marital status, cardiovascular diseases, and cardiovascular risk factors: a review of the evidence. *Journal of Women's Health, 26*(6), 624-632.

29. Chen, B., & Kan, H. (2008). Air pollution and population health: a global challenge. *Environmental health and preventive medicine, 13*, 94-101.

30. Lin, S. (2018). *The Dental Diet: The Surprising Link between Your Teeth, Real Food, and Life-Changing Natural Health.* Hay House.

31. Kloner, R. A., Stanek, E., Desai, K., Crowe, C. L., Paige Ball, K., Haynes, A., & Rosen, R. C. (2024). The association of tadalafil exposure with lower rates of major adverse cardiovascular events and mortality in a general population of men with erectile dysfunction. *Clinical Cardiology, 47*(2), e24234.

Finale: What You Need To Know
By: Jonathan Kahan MD

- Health is not just the absence of disease but about being physically, mentally and emotionally free. Since cardiovascular disease is the #1 cause of mortality and morbidity, it makes sense to focus on this disease category.
- Psst: Smoking is bad for you! To quit, use of nicotine replacement therapy vastly improves outcomes.
- The silent killer: high blood pressure is involved in a multitude of cardiovascular diseases. It responds really well to lifestyle changes and to medications.
    - High cholesterol is correlated with heart attacks and strokes and is less controlled by lifestyle influences than other topics in this book. Certain types of cholesterol plus inflammation lead to plaque formation in the arteries, which is how cardiovascular disease develops. Medications may be considered in this category, know the risks and benefits of each!
- Obesity and metabolic dysfunction lead to inflammation which is the precursor for heart attacks, strokes and death. They are caused by processed foods in the background of lack of exercise/quality sleep. Eating unprocessed foods is the best way to correct this. It is not just about the macros!
- There is no better pill for health than exercise. This is measured by VO2Max. Exercise is broken down into resistance training at least twice a week, base training and high intensity interval training in a 75/25 ratio. Move every day!
- Without quality sleep it is impossible to achieve any of the above metrics. Get light in the morning, avoid stimulants/substances later in the day, no screen time within hours prior to bed, sleep in a cool/dark room.
- Cell phones, screens and social media are the "processed food" of social interaction and removing them from your life is excellent for your overall well-being. Find a purpose higher than yourself, get out in nature, and have real face to face interactions. This is human technology, and it works really well.

Appendix
By: Mohamed Hamed MD, Jonathan Kahan MD

Intervention/ Comparison	Who Delivers It	Who Receives It	Increase in 6-12 Month Abstinence vs no intervention (%)
Brief advice from a doctor vs. no intervention	Doctors	Smokers visiting a clinic	2% (2-3%)
Printed self-help materials vs. nothing	Healthcare providers (like health promotion groups)	Smokers who want help and are ready to quit	2% (1-3%)
Proactive phone support vs. reactive phone support	Trained smoking cessation practitioners	Smokers who want help and are ready to quit	3% (2-4%)
Automated text messaging vs. non-smoking-related messaging	System providers	Smokers who want help and are ready to quit	4% (3-5%)
Face-to-face individual counseling vs. brief advice or written materials	Trained smoking cessation practitioners	Smokers who want help and are ready to quit	4% (3-5%)
Face-to-face group counseling vs. brief advice or written materials	Trained smoking cessation practitioners	Smokers who want help and are ready to quit	5% (4-7%)
Single nicotine replacement therapy (NRT) vs. placebo	Healthcare professionals	Smokers who want help and are ready to quit	6% (6-7%)
Dual form/combination nicotine replacement therapy (NRT) vs. placebo	Healthcare professionals	Smokers who want help and are ready to quit	11%
Cytisine vs. placebo	Healthcare professionals	Smokers who want help and are ready to quit	6% (4-9%)
Bupropion vs. placebo	Healthcare professionals	Smokers who want help and are ready to quit	7% (6-9%)

Nortriptyline vs. placebo	Healthcare professionals	Smokers who want help and are ready to quit	10% (6-15%)
Varenicline vs. placebo	Healthcare professionals	Smokers who want help and are ready to quit	15% (13-17%)

Table 1: Effectiveness of healthcare-based smoking cessation methods, according to Cochrane reviews [11]

	Gum	Lozenge	Transdermal Patch	Nasal Spray	Oral Inhaler
P R O D U C T	Nicorette, Generic OTC 2 mg, 4 mg in original, cinnamon, fruit, mint	Nicorette Lozenge, Nicorette Mini Lozenge, Generic OTC 2 mg, 4 mg in cherry, mint	NicoDerm CQ, Generic OTC 7 mg, 14 mg, 21 mg (24-hour release)	Nicotrol NS Metered spray 10 mg/mL aqueous nicotine solution	Nicotrol Inhaler Rx 10 mg cartridge delivers 4 mg of inhaled nicotine vapor
D O S E	*1st cigarette ≤30 minutes after waking:* 4 mg *1st cigarette >30 minutes after waking:* 2 mg Weeks 1–6: 1 piece q 1–2 hours Weeks 7–9: 1 piece q 2–4 hours Weeks 10–12: 1 piece q 4–8 hours • Maximum, 24 pieces/day • Chew each piece slowly • Park between cheek and gum when peppery or tingling sensation appears (~15–30 chews) • Resume chewing	*1st cigarette ≤30 minutes after waking:* 4 mg *1st cigarette >30 minutes after waking:* 2 mg Weeks 1–6: 1 lozenge q 1–2 hours Weeks 7–9: 1 lozenge q 2–4 hours Weeks 10–12: 1 lozenge q 4–8 hours • Maximum, 20 lozenges/day • Allow to dissolve slowly (20–30 minutes for standard; 10 minutes for mini) • Nicotine release	*>10 cigarettes/day:* 21 mg/day × 4–6 weeks 14 mg/day × 2 weeks 7 mg/day × 2 weeks *≤10 cigarettes/day:* 14 mg/day × 6 weeks 7 mg/day × 2 weeks • May wear patch for 16 hours if patient experiences sleep disturbances (remove at bedtime) • Duration: 8–10 weeks	1–2 doses/hour (8–40 doses/day) One dose ≤ 2 sprays (one in each nostril); each spray delivers 0.5 mg of nicotine to the nasal mucosa • Maximum 5 doses/hour or 40 doses/day • For best results, initially use at least 8 doses/day • Do not sniff, swallow, or inhale	6–16 cartridges/day Individualize dosing; initially use 1 cartridge q 1–2 hours • Best effects with continuous puffing for 20 minutes • Initially use at least 6 cartridges/day • Nicotine in cartridge is depleted after 20 minutes of active puffing • Inhale into back of throat or puff in short breaths • Do NOT inhale into the lungs (like a cigarette) but "puff" as if

139

	• when tingle fades • Repeat chew/park steps until most of the nicotine is gone (tingle does not return; generally 30 min) • Park in different areas of mouth • No food or beverages 15 minutes before or during use • Duration: up to 12 weeks	• may cause a warm, tingling sensation • Do not chew or swallow • Occasionally rotate to different areas of the mouth • No food or beverages 15 minutes before or during use • Duration: up to 12 weeks		• through the nose as the spray is being administered • Duration: 3–6 months	• lighting a pipe • Open cartridge retains potency for 24 hours • No food or beverages 15 minutes before or during use • Duration: 3–6 months
ADVERSE EFFECTS	• Mouth/jaw soreness • Hiccups • Lightheadedness • Nausea	• Nausea • Hiccups • Cough • Heartburn • Headache • Flatulence • Insomnia	• Local skin reactions (erythema, pruritus, burning) • Headache • Sleep disturbances (insomnia, abnormal/vivid dreams); associated with nocturnal nicotine absorption	• Nasal and/or throat irritation (hot, peppery, or burning sensation) • Rhinitis • Tearing • Sneezing • Cough • Headache	• Mouth and/or throat irritation • Cough • Headache • Rhinitis • Dyspepsia • Hiccups
BENEFITS	• Might serve as an oral substitute for tobacco • Might delay weight gain • Can be titrated to manage withdrawal symptoms	• Might serve as an oral substitute for tobacco • Might delay weight gain • Can be titrated to	• Once daily dosing associated with fewer compliance problems • Of all NRT	• Can be titrated to rapidly manage withdrawal symptoms • Can be used in	• Might serve as an oral substitute for tobacco • Can be titrated to manage withdrawal symptoms • Mimics hand-to-mouth

• Can be used in combinatio n with other agents to manage situational urges	manage withdrawal symptoms • Can be used in combinatio n with other agents to manage situational urges	products, its use is least obvious to others • Can be used in combinati on with other agents; delivers consisten t nicotine levels over 24 hours	combin ation with other agents to manage situatio nal urges	ritual of smoking • Can be used in combination with other agents to manage situational urges

Table 2: Nicotine Replacement Therapy (NRT) Formulations [6, smoking chapter]

Lipid pathway expanded:

How cholesterol/triglycerides are processed in the body:

1. Cholesterol and triglycerides enter our bodies by eating food. In terms of mass, triglycerides outweigh cholesterol 10-100x in animal products. Note plants do not have cholesterol but do have triglycerides. We can also make cholesterol and make triglycerides from excess sugar/carbohydrate intake in the liver.

2. Triglycerides are further classified into monounsaturated (aka omega 9), polyunsaturated (omega 3,6), saturated, or trans fats. These, and cholesterols, are broken down by stomach acids into smaller droplets called emulsified fats where they travel to the small intestine.

3. In the small intestine, bile acids from the liver surround the emulsified fat droplets. Triglycerides (TGs) have an extra step and are further broken down into fatty acids and monoglycerides by the pancreatic enzyme lipase (-ase always denotes an enzyme which is a protein that performs a chemical reaction).

4. These components are then repackaged across the small intestine into spheres of triglycerides/cholesterols within an apolipoprotein (protein) cage called a chylomicron. Once

formed, the chylomicron goes from the small intestine cells into the lymphatic system then it gets dumped via the thoracic duct into the bloodstream.

5. From there the chylomicrons go down the bloodstream into the tiny capillaries that are beside muscle and adipose (fat) cells. A receptor called Lipoprotein Lipase (LPL) takes up the free fatty acids (from TGs) to be used in energy or storage for later in the case of muscle cells and in the case of fat cells they are recombined with glycerol to form triglycerides again for storage in vacuoles (giant balloons for fat storage).

6. The result of this offloading of TG is the creation of a chylomicron remnant that contains a lot more cholesterol and a lot less TG. This then goes to the liver where the cholesterol is taken up by the LDL Receptor and Remnant Receptor-1 (note the chylomicron does not have LDL in it, it has undifferentiated cholesterol).

    a. Note the liver can make its own cholesterol and triglycerides.

7. In the liver, the cholesterols and remaining triglycerides are processed and can become several things:

    a. They can become bile acids which can be used to absorb more cholesterol/triglycerides (see above).

    b. They can become High Density Lipoprotein (HDL) particles, which go to other tissues to bring back cholesterols for repackaging or excretion by the liver. The main protein surrounding this core of liquid cholesterol is apolipoprotein A-I (apoA-I).

    c. They can become Very Low-Density Lipoprotein (VLDL) particles. These are spherical mixtures of cholesterols, TGs and phospholipids all surrounded by apolipoprotein B (apoB). The VLDL particles then go to muscle and adipose cells via the bloodstream where they (again) dump TG into these cells via the LpL receptor (again) and the VLDL becomes an LDL (low density lipoprotein) which is loaded with cholesterol. Note LDL is made in the bloodstream, not liver. The LDL then goes and gives cholesterol to various cells to make cell membranes, steroids etc.

i. Note also that the same apoB protein surrounds all the LDL, VLDL and IDL (the short lived intermediate between VLDL and LDL particles).

ii. Once the LDL particles have offloaded their TG and cholesterol, they return to the liver where they can become Lp(a) or be reprocessed into a.b. or c.

d. Lp(a) (lipoprotein "little" a): these small LDL (surrounded by apoB) particles can come back to the liver after giving most of its cholesterol, where an apoa protein tail is attached to the outside of the apoB, making it the most atherogenic particle. This process is entirely genetically driven. See below for a whole section on Lp(a)

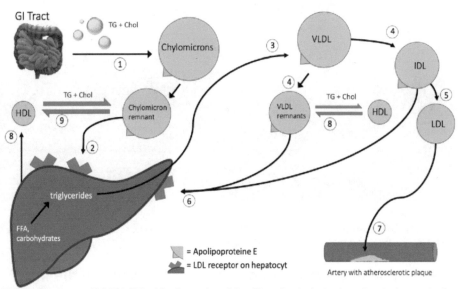

Reeg, Susanne. (2020). What is the role of ApoE variants in ischemic stroke and other age-related complex diseases? 10.13140/RG.2.2.23487.79529.

B. How the processing of cholesterol/triglycerides results in plaque formation.

8. The apoB protein (which contains VLDL, IDL, LDL) or Lp(a) (which is the apoB protein, with small amounts of LDL cholesterol and an extra tail) circulate in the bloodstream and become stuck in the walls of the arteries. This triggers a

reaction where these particles get oxidized by reactive oxygen species (ROS). ROS can be smoke inhalation, UV exposure, free radicals etc.

9. When apoB or Lp(a) proteins become oxidized the body attacks them with immune cells called macrophages, which eat the oxidized lipid particles and become foam cells, triggering an inflammation cascade and grow to form plaques in the arteries of our body. This process begins when we are about 8 years old!

10. These plaques are unstable and are in the constant process of "exploding and remodeling". For example, a plaque doesn't go from 98%, 99% then 100% and a patient has a heart attack, it goes from 20-30%, then to 70%, then back down to 60%, then 100% and a patient grabs his chest while having a myocardial infarction.

11. **We are done! Jeez!**

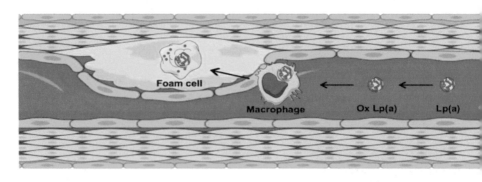

Ugovšek S, Šebeštjen M. Lipoprotein(a)—The Crossroads of Atherosclerosis, Atherothrombosis and Inflammation. *Biomolecules.* 2022; 12(1):26. https://doi.org/10.3390/biom12010026

C. Not so fast! What about cholesterol synthesis in the liver?

In the liver, cholesterol starts with the production of HGM-CoA, whose creation is halted by the statin class of medications. Once cholesterol is made it is then packaged into the VLDL and then converted into LDL in the bloodstream by the same mechanisms above or converted into bile acids. This whole process is regulated by dietary intake, internal controls, hormones, genetics to ensure the body has adequate supplies of all forms of cholesterol.

What is the new AHA prevention calculator?

PREVENT™ Online Calculator

Welcome to the American Heart Association **Predicting Risk of cardiovascular disease EVENTs** (PREVENT™). This app should be used for primary prevention patients (those without atherosclerotic cardiovascular disease or heart failure) only.

Sex	◉ Male ○ Female

Age

| 30-79 | years |

Total Cholesterol

| 130-320 | mg/dL |

HDL Cholesterol

| 20-100 | mg/dL |

SBP

| 90-200 | mmHg |

BMI

| 18.5-39.9 | |

eGFR

| 15-140 | |

Diabetes	◉ No ○ Yes
Current Smoking	◉ No ○ Yes
Anti-hypertensive medication	◉ No ○ Yes
Lipid-lowering medication	◉ No ○ Yes

The following three predictors are optional for further personalization of risk assessment. When

Khan, S. S., Matsushita, K., Sang, Y., Ballew, S. H., Grams, M. E., Surapaneni, A., ... & Chronic Kidney Disease Prognosis Consortium and the American Heart Association Cardiovascular-Kidney-Metabolic Science Advisory Group. (2024). Development and Validation of the American Heart Association's PREVENT Equations. *Circulation*, *149*(6), 430-449.

What labs do we routinely order?

Lab Category	Lab	Logic
Hematology	Complete blood count, iron profile, B12/folate, homocysteine	Assess hematologic function, cause of multitude of diseases. Assess inflammation as well.
Liver/Kidney /Electrolytes	Comprehensive metabolic profile	Includes liver, kidney, nutritional status and electrolytes in one test
Thyroid	TSH and Free T4	Assess thyroid function
Cholesterol	Lipid profile, apolipoprotein B, Lp(a), high sensitivity CRP, sed rate, uric acid.	See cholesterol chapter, checks for lipids and inflammation.
Sugars	HbA1c and fasting insulin	Checks for metabolic syndrome preDM, DM and HOMA-IR calculation.
Magnesium and Vitamin	Magnesium and Vit D 25-OH	Always a separate blood test. See supplement chapter

D		
Hormones	Patient Dependent	Depending on the clinical context, talk to your physician.

Note this is not an exhaustive list and is highly patient dependent, talk to your health care provider.

Basic Biostatistics Definitions
By: Mohamed Hamed MD, Jonathan Kahan MD

What you need to know

We included this very brief section to explain some of the different statistics seen in research papers in a very basic way. This is how you will know the effect size of a particular treatment or be able to evaluate the data yourself. This is not an exhaustive list and it can get quite complicated.

Median

It is the central number of a data set. For example, in the data set of 1,2,5,6 and 7 the median is 5

Mean

It is the average value of the data set. For example, in the data set 1,3,5,8 and 9 (1+2+5+6+7=15, 21/5 = 4.2) the average is 4.2.

Incidence

It is the rate or occurrence of new events in a certain population over a specific period of time. For example, the incidence of people in the United States who have a heart attack per year is about 805,000 people/year.

Prevalence

It is the proportion of a certain population that is affected by a certain condition at a specific time. For example, the prevalence of coronary heart disease in the United States is about 20.5 million people.

Odds ratio (OR)

It is a measure of how strongly an event is associated with exposure.

For example: Odds ratio is 20 for smoking causing lung cancer. This means that hypothetically a smoker has 20 times the odds of having lung cancer.

Relative risk (RR)

It is the probability of an outcome in an exposed group to the probability of an outcome in an unexposed group.

For example: If relative risk is 18, this means that smokers are 18 times likely to develop lung cancer than non-smokers.

Hazard ratio (HR)

It is a measure of how often a particular event happens in one group compared to how often it happens in another group, over a period of time.

For example: The hazard ratio for certain drug is 0.60 that means that the study drug provides 40% risk reduction compared to the control group.

Number needed to harm (NNH)

The number of people that are exposed to something that causes harm to one person. E.g. a NNH of 7 means one person is harmed for every 7 people exposed.

Number needed to treat (NTT)

The number of people that are needed to be treated for one of them to benefit compared to the control group. a NNT of 7 means one person is treated for every 7 people exposed.

Confidence interval (CI)

It is a way to describe probability, it describes an estimate to fall between if you redo your test with a certain level of confidence. Usually the 95% confidence interval is used which means you have a 5% chance of being wrong. It usually has lower and upper endpoints. If the CI crosses 0 or 1 then the observation was not significant. For example, the average height of a 16 years old has 95% CI (5'4", 5'9"). This means that we are confident 95% that their height falls in this range. Another example is say a 95% CI is (0.2-7). This means that it is not a significant result since the confidence interval crosses one.

P- Value

It is used to measure the probability that an observed difference might have occurred by random chance. In medicine it is significant when it is less than 0.05, which means less than 5% chance that a study result was seen based on random chance.

For example, p-value 0.025 means that there is 2.5% chance of the results being random or happened by chance.

Made in the USA
Columbia, SC
07 June 2024

36822161R00083